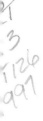

Teaching in the Community

PREPARING NURSES FOR THE 21ST CENTURY

Edited by

M. Elaine Tagliareni

and

Barbara B. Marckx

National League for Nursing Press • New York
Pub. No. 14-7262

Teaching in the community : preparing nurses for the 21st century /
    edited by M. Elaine Tagliareni & Barbara Marckx
        p.   cm.
    "Pub. no. 14-7262."
    Includes bibliographical references and index.
    ISBN 0-88737-726-2
    1. Nursing—Study and teaching.   2. Community health nursing—
Study and teaching.   I. Tagliareni, M. Elaine.   II. Marckx,
Barbara.
RT73.T345   1997
610.73'0711—dc21   97-11195
                                                                                 CIP

This book was set in 11 point Goudy by Publications Development Company of Texas. The designer was Allan Graubard. The printer was Bookcrafters. The cover was designed by Lauren Stevens.

Printed in the United States of America

Contributors List

Bonnie L. Ashcroft, MS, RN
Former Project Director,
Rural Nursing Centers Project
Penn State School of Nursing
University Park, Pennsylvania

Evelyn C. Atchison, EdD, RN
Program Head, Nursing
Northern Virginia Community College
Annandale, Virginia

Elaine Bower, MSN, RN
Assistant Professor
Community College of Philadelphia
Philadelphia, Pennsylvania

Marjorie Buchanan, MSN, RN
Executive Assistant to the President
Independence Foundation
Philadelphia, Pennsylvania

Mary Capozzi, MS, RN
Chairperson
Nursing Department
Finger Lakes Community College
Canandaigua, New York

Michelle Codner, RN, MS
Clinical Instructor, Maternal-Child
    Nursing
Department of Nursing
Broome Community College
Binghamton, New York

Ivory Coleman, MSN, RN
Professor, Nursing
Community College of Philadelphia
Philadelphia, Pennsylvania

Geraldine C. Colombraro, RN, MA,
    PhD (Candidate)
Assistant Dean
Center for Continuing Education in
    Nursing and Health Care
Leinhard School of Nursing
Pace University
Pleasantville, New York

Charlene Connolly, EdD, RN, CHES
Chair
Health Technologies Division
Northern Virginia Community College
Annandale, Virginia

Karin Conway, RN, BSN
Director of Business Operations and
    Care Environment
Columbia Home Care
Denver, Colorado

Janet Z. Denman, MS, RN
Associate Professor
Broome Community College
Binghamton, New York

Ruth A. DePalma RN, MSN
Assistant Professor of Nursing/Nursing
    Services Coordinator
University of Southern Colorado/
    Pueblo School District 60
Pueblo, Colorado

Gloria Donnelly, PhD, RN, FAAN
Dean, School of Nursing
Allegheny University
Philadelphia, Pennsylvania

Kelly Gallant, RN, BSN
Homecare Supervisor
Columbia Home Care
Denver, Colorado

Clare T. Garrard, RN, BSN, MSN, DSN
Associate Professor of Nursing
Floyd College
Rome, Georgia

Mary Anne Gauthier, EdD, RN
Associate Professor
College of Nursing
Northeastern University
Boston, Massachusetts

Mary Beth Hanner, PhD, RN
Dean of Nursing Programs
Regents College
The University of the State of New York
Albany, New York

Jean Haspeslagh, DNS, RN
Associate Professor
School of Nursing
University of Southern Mississippi
Hattiesburg, Mississippi

Joan E. Henshaw, RN, MS
Professor of Nursing
Front Range Community College,
    Westminster Campus
Westminster, Colorado

Stephen Paul Holzemer, PhD, RN
Dean
School of Nursing
The Long Island College Hospital
School of Nursing
Brooklyn, New York

Susan Johnson, EdD, MPH, CPNP, RN
Chairperson
Department of Nursing
University of South Dakota
Vermillion, South Dakota

Barbara Kelley, EdD, RN, MPH, CPNP
Assistant Professor
College of Nursing
Northeastern University
Boston, Massachusetts

June Larson, MSN, RN
Director
Department of Nursing in Vermillion
University of South Dakota
Vermillion, South Dakota

Margaret Ann Mahoney, PhD, RN
Assistant Professor
College of Nursing
Northeastern University
Boston, Massachusetts

Ann Marie LaMarca Major, MS,
    RNC, CS
Clinical Instructor
Decker School of Nursing
Binghamton University
Binghamton, New York

Barbara B. Marckx, MS, RN
Professor of Nursing
Broome Community College
Binghamton, New York

Peggy S. Matteson, PhD, RNC
Assistant Professor
College of Nursing
Northeastern University
Boston, Massachusetts

Barbara Mc Laughlin, MSN, RN
Assistant Professor
Community College of Philadelphia
Philadelphia, Pennsylvania

Andrea Mengel, PhD, RN
Professor and Head
Nursing Department
Community College of Philadelphia
Philadelphia, Pennsylvania

Alma L. Mueller, RN, MEd
Program Director and Professor of
    Nursing
Front Range Community College,
    Westminster Campus
Westminster, Colorado

Heather Reece-Tillack, MS, RN
Instructor of Nursing
Finger Lakes Community College
Canandiagua, New York

Susan Sherman, MA, RN
President
Independence Foundation
Philadelphia, Pennsylvania

Susan Stocker, MSN, RN
Assistant Professor
Kent State University
Ashtabula, Ohio

Carol Stuart, MSN, RN
Director
Department of Nursing in Sioux Falls
University of South Dakota
Vermillion, South Dakota

M. Elaine Tagliareni, MS, RN
Associate Professor, Nursing
Independence Chair
Community Health Nursing Education
Community College of Philadelphia
Philadelphia, Pennsylvania

Vicky Talbert, MS, RN-C, PNP
Clinical Assistant Professor
School of Nursing
University of Wisconsin-Milwaukee
Milwaukee, Wisconsin

Linda L. Vance, PhD
Former Director of Planning and
    Development, Home Health Agency
Community Consultant on Strategic
    Planning, Program Assessment and
    Development
Penn State University
University Park, Pennsylvania

Jacqueline Watercutter, MS, RN
Assistant Professor
Edison Community College
Piqua, Ohio

Barbara White, RN, BSN, MS
Assistant Professor
Department of Nursing
Regis University
Denver, Colorado

Joan Wilk, PhD, RN
Associate Professor
School of Nursing
University of Wisconsin-Milwaukee
Milwaukee, Wisconsin

Elizabeth Windstein, MS, RN
Community Health Instructor
Finger Lakes Community College
Canandiagua, New York

Sue A. Wise, MS, RN, CSW
Assistant Professor
Edison Community College
Piqua, Ohio

Susan C. Youtz, MA, RN
Assistant Director
Penn State School of Nursing
University Park, Pennsylvania

Contents

Foreword

Every nursing faculty today, regardless of the type of program, faces a herculean task: The nursing curriculum must be refocused and restructured for a health care world that is no longer predictable. (It may never have been predictable, but at least it seemed so.) Furthermore, the challenge to the faculty is not, as once thought, to develop an educational program which anticipates the future while adhering to a known present, but instead to see both present and future practice of RNs as essentially undefined. *Teaching in the Community* suggests how nursing faculty might make way in their thinking for creative, flexible curricula, envisioning a new landscape and new ways of viewing and organizing the student experience. This book offers inspiring accounts of a number of ways in which a faculty can succeed in achieving change in the teaching-learning transactions. There are others, perhaps as many as the number of faculties who take up the challenge of refocusing and restructuring the curriculum to prepare nurses for the 21st century.

Books such as this one with chapters written by authors allied with associate, baccalaureate, and graduate programs signal a new era of collaboration and cooperation among nursing educators. The change of focus from alienating adversarial criticism and needless rivalry to the collaboration represented here is refreshing and revitalizing. Nursing practice and education must change radically in order to be able to respond effectively to society's needs. The scope of change requires the talents and strengths of all educators working together. This book does not address differentiation among types of programs, an overworked approach belonging to the past. It puts the focus on the significant concerns of all of nursing today and will require our best and closest joint efforts to manage nursing education's course in today's fluid and uncertain health care environment.

The coming new millennium prompts thoughts of change and new be-ginnings. We believe nursing educators must bring an end to educational practices that have served us with varying degrees of success in these closing decades of the 20th century so that we will herald the dawn of the 21st with an awakened sense of unity and a determination to achieve the goals of community-based nursing. This fine book offers guidelines for setting forth.

VERLE WATERS

EM OLIVIA BEVIS

Preface

This book is about innovation, new ideas, and thinking differently about nursing education and practice in a reformed health care system for the 21st century. The ideas and projects presented reflect the collective expertise of nursing faculty nationally who have accepted ambiguity, diverged from traditional educational models, and ventured forth into unchartered venues.

As nurse educators began to place students in community settings, especially nursing homes and long-term care facilities, it became evident that students at every level of education could find meaningful learning experiences in such care environments. Beyond the traditional fundamental tasks were also higher order activities that stimulated the students' creativity and resourcefulness. Simultaneously, as nurse educators were responding to guidelines for future health practice as developed by national organizations, they realized how necessary it was to broaden such response into imperatives for the curriculum itself.

During the past several years as well, we have experienced a groundswell of interest by nurse educators in exploring innovative approaches to teaching in the community. Faculty from all levels of nursing education seek to move beyond traditional definitions of community nursing practice, which have been limited historically to home care. The commitment to adopt a broader scope of community-based nursing began to flourish.

Thus, as editors, we have worked to provide a resource and guidebook to help nursing educators revise curriculum, expand community nursing content, and develop clinical teaching opportunities that are community-based. We have attempted to provide a wide spectrum of teaching approaches from both associate and baccalaurate nurse educators, representing diverse communities from across the country.

The book is organized to move the reader from broad educational concepts about community practice and faculty role changes to specific examples of innovative curriculum models and individual community-based projects. Because we believe that the health care professional of the future will need to work effectively in collaborative relationships with peers and interdisciplinary colleagues, a section of the book is devoted to creating complementary paths within nursing and with other health care professionals.

The nursing educators who have contributed to this volume are committed to advances in nursing education, and we applaud them for the time they devoted to complete chapters, against short deadlines. Our thanks also go to Susan Sherman, President, Independence Foundation, Philadelphia, Pennsylvania., and Linda Crawford, Associate Director for the Center for Research, NLN. Without their initiative and vision, this project would never have been launched. A special thank you to Allan Graubard, Director, NLN Press, and his staff who worked closely with us, over many months, to bring this book to completion.

Although neither of us came to this endeavor with a background in community health nursing, like so many nurse educators nationally, we bring a commitment to the future direction of health care and to the successful movement of fellow nursing educators to a zone of comfort in the uncertain and fluid environment of the community. Our vision for nursing education is one of collaboration and connections. Ironically, as we collaborated on author selection and manuscript development while editing this volume, we uncovered personal and professional connections about ourselves that facilitated our working relationship. We are both graduates of Georgetown University School of Nursing and have made a lifetime commitment to associate degree nursing education; both of us also have two wonderful children and loving and supportive husbands. We hope that our book will assist and encourage you, our nursing colleagues, to discover similar connections both within our profession and our communities.

M. Elaine Tagliareni
Barbara B. Marckx

SECTION I

Thinking Differently about Nursing Education and Practice

1

The New System of Care

Nursing and Health

Marjorie Buchanan

The greatest thing in this world is not so much where we are, but in what direction we are moving.

Oliver Wendell Holmes

Health is a resource for everyday life. Family, work, and other responsibilities require levels of energy, fitness, and overall hardiness that enable people to meet their responsibilities, carry out their daily tasks, and engage in meaningful activities. Toward that end, a long overdue shift is taking place in the professional health care system—a focus on *health* rather than *illness* care. Individual and institutional providers alike are moving beyond crisis intervention and medical treatment, and actively incorporating health promotion and protection services into the care continuum. The interrelationship between socioeconomic status and health status is more readily acknowledged. Linkages between poverty and high rates of both chronic and communicable disease, cultural differences and limited access to care, urban problems or rural isolation that may limit availability of services, and other factors are gaining long overdue recognition by both providers and policymakers. Organizational, regulatory, and financing mechanisms are gradually realigning themselves with these factors in mind.

The single most driving force in this era of health care reorientation is the rapid upward spiral of medical care costs to consumers, employers and third-party payers such as traditional private insurers, managed care

3

organizations, and the government programs of Medicare and Medicaid. The broader costs of preventable health problems to society must also be noted. Increasing incidence and prevalence of communicable and chronic diseases (once on the decline), newly emerging catastrophic communicable diseases, decreased productivity in the workplace by both those who are ill and their caregivers, increased family dependency on social support services, and many other issues challenge the abilities of the health care system and communities to thrive.

This chapter presents an overview of the changing health care environment with the challenges and opportunities it poses for the nursing profession. Within the context of health care reform in the United States over time, information is shared about building a comprehensive, effective and affordable primary health care system devised in partnership with the community, based in the community, and focused on the community.

NURSING AND HEALTH: A CHALLENGE
TO THE PROFESSION

The roles, responsibilities, and educational preparation of health care providers from all disciplines have been carefully scrutinized in light of this emerging awareness of the complex factors influencing health and health care. Recommendations from The Pew Health Professions Commissions, The National League for Nursing, the U.S. Public Health Service Bureau of Health Professions and others (Larson, 1995) convey a mandate for change in both health care and health professionals' education to ensure that people have what is needed to be healthy and to reduce the overwhelming costs of care to the nation (see Table 1–1).

After decades of working in a biomedical model that is disease-focused, oriented to individuals, and organized around providers rather than those they serve, nursing is somewhat poorly positioned to meet the challenges and opportunities that lie ahead. Health policy, financial mechanisms for health care, organizational structure, and attitudinal barriers have obstructed the public's direct accessing of nursing services committed to health and caring. Knowledge and skills in health promotion and disease prevention, in community-based and community-focused care, and in multisector community collaboration will need to be honed to achieve full participation in the shift toward health-focused care.

Table 1–1
Recent Recommendations for
Health Care Professional Reform

Organization	Recommendations
Pew Charitable Trusts' **Health Professions Commission** *Health Professions Education for the Future: Schools in Service to the Nation.* February 1993.	• Build from a foundation of values. • Concentrate on core educational activities. • Redefine political and economic relationships. • Focus on the health needs of the community. • Strengthen tools for change.
U.S. Department of Health and Human Services' **Bureau of Health Professions** *An Agenda for Health Professions Reform.* February 1993.	• Promote primary care education. • Strengthen and expand public health education and practice. • Expand the capacity of nursing and allied health professions to meet the increasing demand for services. • Increase numbers of health care providers from minority/disadvantaged backgrounds. • Promote educational strategies to recruit and retain health care providers from underserved populations. • Advance continuous quality improvement in health promotions education and practice. • Strengthen health professions data, information systems, and education research.
Alliance for Health Reform *Commanding Generalists: Increasing the Availability of Community-Based Primary Care Practitioners.* July 1993.	• Change health professional schools' admission policies. • Modify health professional schools' curriculum and environment to give students primary care experiences in community settings, increase understanding of behavioral and social components of health and illness, ensure exposure to multidisciplinary teams. • Increase supply of nurse practitioners, nurse midwives, physician assistants, and others. • Retrain specialists as generalists.

(Continued)

Table 1–1 (**Continued**)

Organization	Recommendations
American Association of Colleges of Nursing *Nursing Education's Agenda for the 21st Century.* March 1993.	• Comprehensive review of mission for relevance to health care needs. • Organizational structure that facilitates new initiatives. • Redefine faculty scholarship to include practice. • Recruitment and retention of a diverse student body. • Emphasize curricular processes that develop critical thinking, ethical decision-making, interdisciplinary participation, coordination. • Curriculum content should include health promotion and maintenance; economics; ethical, legal, political principles; and informatics. • Program evaluation and outcomes are integral to the curriculum. • Enhance integration of nursing research into schools and the mainstream scientific community.
National League for Nursing *A Vision for Nursing Education.* June 1993.	• Rethink mission of nursing education to promote quality for care and to create linkages for service. • Increasingly plan educational experiences when people are home, at school, or work, or receiving long-term care, etc. • Curricular reform to match needs of health care environment; and to focus on processes such as critical thinking, shared decision-making collaboration. • Faculty reform to focus on the scholarship of application.

Note: From "New Rules for the Game: Interdisciplinary Education for Health Professionals," by E. Larson, 1995, *Nursing Outlook.* July/August.

The profession must move quickly to refocus its notions about practice, education, and research. Practicing nurses must retool for noninstitutional roles and responsibilities. Nursing faculty must reflect on and redesign nursing education to adequately prepare new practitioners for their roles in this reconfigured health care system. Nurse researchers must examine nursing's impact on health status through careful examination of the relationships among content and quality of care, access to care, and cost of care.

HISTORICAL OVERVIEW OF HEALTH CARE REFORM

Although health care reform is often conveyed as a current phenomenon, reform efforts are continuous, each emerging from preceding decades of social concern, health information, research and development, and public policy changes. Each era reflects its own concerns, issues, tensions, questions, doubts, visions, courage, and creativity. Successes, breakthroughs, mistakes, and midcourse corrections occur, yielding to the next phase of reform (see Table 1–2).

It is possible to gain insight into the current state of health affairs by looking back over time. Greater understanding of disease causation and transmission led to sanitation and communicable disease control in the late 1800s and early 1900s. Medical care developments during World War II yielded postwar development in scientific knowledge, medical facilities, and health personnel. An infrastructure emerged with a biomedical orientation to care rather than health. As institutional care rose, community care diminished. Later, social concerns about lack of access to many of these resources by the poor and elderly led to public policy developments in the form of Medicare, Medicaid, and the establishment of neighborhood health centers (Green & Kreuter, 1991).

Rising costs of care, continuing socioeconomic and racial disparities, and only marginal improvements in overall health status raised concerns. Public questions were posed about the continuing focus on highly technological care with its increasing costs for medical services. In the early 1970s, the cost of care began to overwhelm health insurers, business and industry, and government. Efforts at cost containment were undertaken through such initiatives as diagnosis-related group (DRG) protocols for service use and the creation of health maintenance organizations (HMOs). These efforts, however, did not adequately address such key issues as the aging of the population, rising rates of preventable chronic and communicable disease and other conditions. The need to redirect health care priorities, policies and financing mechanisms toward a health model of care became increasingly apparent. (Green & Kreuter, 1991).

Table 1–2
Eras of Health Care Reform

Era	Focus	Key Outcomes
1800–1900	Communicable Disease	• Sanitation and environmental health.
1900–1945	Infections and Trauma	• Health departments (case finding and quarantine). • Safe hospitals. • Advances in surgery/childbirth. • Discoveries of disease causation and treatments (antibiotics, insulin).
Post World War II: 1940s and 1950s	Resource Development	• Biomedical infrastructure (hospitals, research, manpower). • Emerging questions about equitable distribution.
1960s and 1970s	Redistribution of Resources	• Medicare/Medicaid. • Neighborhood health centers. • Greater access, although continued disparity. • Emerging questions about unnecessary/excessive services.
1980s	Cost Containment	• DRGs. • HMOs. • Public health education. • Self-care education. • Emerging questions about rising rates of preventable chronic disease.
1990s	Health Promotion Policy	• Shared responsibility. • Multisector collaboration. • Lifestyle construct for health. • Multilevel intervention.

Note: From *Health Promotion Planning: An Educational and Environmental Approach,* by L. Green and M. Kreuter, 1991, (p. xxx), Mountain View, California: Mayfield Publishing Co.

In 1948, the World Health Organization defined "health as a state of complete physical, mental and social well-being and not merely the absence of disease." Affirmed at the 1978 Alma Eta Conference of WHO in what was then the USSR, nations updated that definition, stating that health is "a state of enough physical, mental, and social well-being to enable people to work productively and participate actively in the social and economic life of the community in which they live." They noted the importance of full and organized community participation and ultimate self-reliance, with individuals, families, and communities assuming more responsibility for their own health. Commitments were made by all nations to strive for *primary health care* for all by the year 2000 (Anderson & McFarlane, 1996).

The primary health care model comprised elements and priorities beyond the professional health care system (Figure 1–1). Full implementation of this model will require a shifting of services and resources to more fully support primary care and self-health care in the home and community, rather than concentrating them in the secondary and tertiary care arenas (see Table 1–3).

The United States lags behind other nations in moving toward this goal. The focus on biomedical technology and the institutionalization

Figure 1–1
Primary Health Care Model

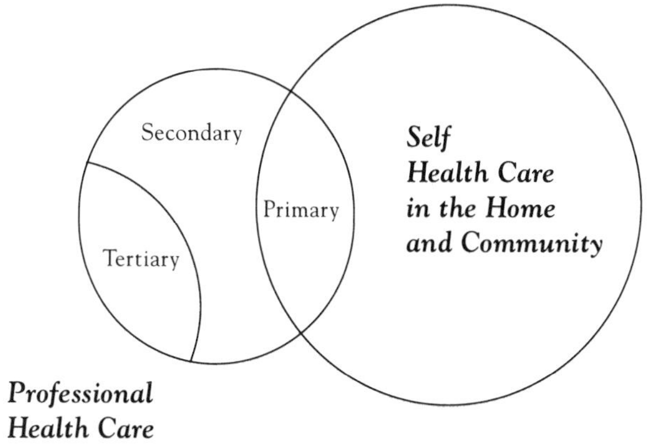

Note: Adapted from "Primary Health Care: An Answer to the Dilemmas of Community Nursing" by J. Goeppinger, 1984, *Nursing Outlook 1*(3), pp. 129–140. Copyright 1984 by Mosby-Year Book, Inc.. Used with permission.

Table 1–3
Primary Health Care (WHO, 1978)

Definition	• Is essential health care. • Based on practical, scientifically sound and socially acceptable methods and technology. • Universally accessible to all in the community through their full participation. • At an affordable cost. • Geared toward self-reliance and self-determination.
Integration into the Health Care System and the Community	• Forms an integral part of both the health system and . . . the overall social and economic development of the community. • Is the main focus and central function of the health system. • Is the first level of contact of people with the health system. • Health care is as close as possible to where people live and work. • Constitutes the first element of a continuing health process.
Essential Concepts in Ensuring Health Care for All	• Maximum involvement of people in their own health care and the development of their self reliance. • Involvement and cooperation of persons and agencies from many sectors (safety and transportation, communications, and so forth). • Use of scientifically sound technologies that are appropriate, acceptable, and affordable. • Availability of essential medicines.
Priorities for Action	1. Education for the identification and prevention/control of prevailing health problems. 2. Proper food supplies and nutrition. 3. Adequate supply of safe water and basic sanitation. 4. Maternal and child care, including family planning. 5. Immunization against the major infectious diseases; prevention and control of locally endemic diseases. 6. Appropriate treatment of common diseases using appropriate technology. 7. Promotion of mental health. 8. Provision of essential drugs.

Note: From *Community as Partner* by E. Anderson and J. McFarlane, 1996, Philadelphia: Lippincott-Raven.

of the health care system after World War II are the major reasons for this situation. The present attention on health promotion and disease prevention provides an opportunity to change this situation. By shifting from a health care paradigm focused on illness to one focused on health, the primary health care model can be fully implemented (see Figure 1–2).

In 1995, a useful diagram was developed as part of the U.S. Public Health Service *Core Functions Project* illustrating that population-based public health programs focusing on health protection, disease prevention, and health promotion provide the foundation on which primary secondary and tertiary care rest (Figure 1–3). All levels of care are important to the health of the population and thus must be part of a health-oriented care system, but "the greater the effectiveness of services in the lower tiers, the greater is the capability of higher tiers to contribute efficiently to health improvement" (U.S. Public Health Service, 1995).

Recommendations that emerged from the *Core Functions Project* focus on committing greater attention and resources on population-based health care services, clinical preventive services, and primary health care and reducing the requirements for higher levels of care.

Figure 1–2
Paradigm Shift

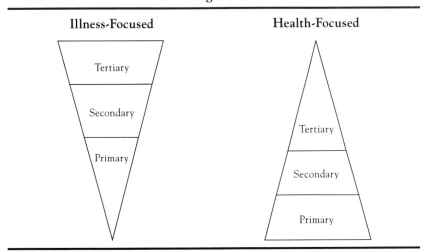

Illness-Focused

Tertiary
Secondary
Primary

Health-Focused

Tertiary
Secondary
Primary

Figure 1–3
Health Services Pyramid

Core Functions Project, U.S. Public Health Service

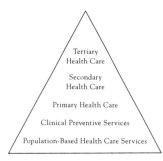

Tertiary
Health Care

Secondary
Health Care

Primary Health Care

Clinical Preventive Services

Population-Based Health Care Services

The greater the effectiveness of services in the lower tiers, the greater is the capability of higher tiers to contribute efficiently to health improvements.

—*U. S. Prevention Report,* 1995

Population-Based Health Care Services	Problems are defined (diagnoses) and solutions (interventions) are proposed for defined populations or subpopulations, as opposed to diagnoses and intervention/treatment carried out at an individual patient or client level.
Clinical Preventive Services	*Primary Prevention:* Actions that reduce the incidence of disease by promoting health and preventing the development of disease processes (e.g. immunization, diet and exercise).
	Secondary Prevention: Programs such as screening, designed to detect disease in the early stages (early pathogenesis) before clinically evident signs and symptoms, in order to intervene with early diagnosis and treatment. (e.g., Pap smear, HIV screening, mammography).
Primary Health Care	Public health and primary care services; it includes delivering essential, affordable, accessible, and acceptable health care to the community, with an emphasis on disease prevention and health promotion, community involvement, multisectoral cooperation and appropriate technology.
	Primary Care: Typically, the entry point into the health care delivery system; emphasizes the management of commonly occurring diseases or chronic disease.
Secondary Health Care	Actions to treat disease in its early acute phase; services arranged through referral or consultation after a preliminary evaluation by a primary-care practitioner.
	Services available at most community hospitals; include most surgery and such medical specialties as radiologists, cardiologists and endocrinologists.
Tertiary Health Care	Actions taken to limit the progression of disease or disability.
	Highly specialized diagnostic, therapeutic and rehabilitative services requiring staff and equipment of a major medical center.

HEALTH PROMOTION AND PROTECTION

Primary health care incorporates the notion of health as a resource for everyday life. Embedded in an array of factors that contribute to people's overall quality of life, health care involves much more than health status considerations of mortality, morbidity, and *length* of life. Quality of life also includes life satisfaction, personal and social resources, stressful life events, employment rates, housing density, air quality, and myriad other factors (Figure 1–4).

Relationships between health and social conditions are reciprocal and thus must be considered in tandem. *Health promotion* is the broad concept that seeks to increase the physical, social and emotional health and well-being of individuals, families, and communities. Terms such as high-level wellness, fitness, hardiness refer to optimal levels of health as defined within both personal and community contexts, and by population-based standards. Efforts focus primarily on health education and the establishment of necessary environmental conditions and resources for health. Behaviors related to nutrition, mental health, physical activity and fitness, family planning, violent and abusive behavior, and consumption of tobacco, alcohol, and other drugs all are addressed through educational and community-based programs.

Health protection is one aspect of health promotion focusing on environmental health, occupational safety and health, accidental unintentional injuries, food and drug safety, oral health, and other elements that pose a threat to people in their daily lives. Elements not previously considered health problems per se, such as domestic and community violence, are increasingly being incorporated into the health protection domain. *Disease*

Figure 1–4
Health Status Contributes to a Person's Quality of Life

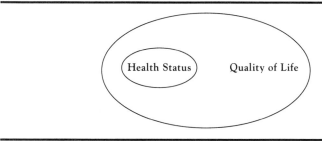

prevention, in turn, is one aspect of health protection. Disease prevention efforts focus on maternal and infant health care, immunizations and infectious diseases, chronic disease, and physically and mentally disabling disorders and conditions.

For many years, efforts were directed at changing lifestyles and behaviors through health programs and activities directed at individuals and families. However, the desired improvements in health status often require more pervasive changes. Ensuring that essential resources and environmental conditions for health are in place requires decision-making and action by communities and the broader social and political systems and structures at local, state, and federal levels. Awareness and information about health and primary health care must occur at all levels to ensure that the necessary resources for health are available and accessible to those most in need of them. Improved family health through lifestyle changes and other forms of self-care can come about only if educational and service programs are in place. Communities, health care providers, and others can only offer such services if policies, regulatory mechanisms and funding streams are in place to support such efforts. Therefore, multilevel intervention is required to bring about needed health care changes (Figure 1–5).

Figure 1–5
Multilevel Intervention*

Individuals
and
Families

Community

Sociopolitical Systems
and Structures

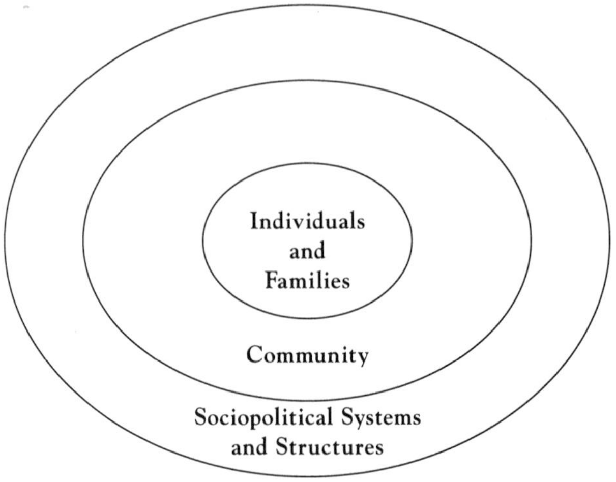

* All who affect and are affected by health care change.

COMMUNITY HEALTH CARE

As the care system begins to shift toward health, more and more services are moving outside their institutional homes and into the communities where people live and work. Transportation, cultural and language differences, environmental issues that have long served as barriers to care are greatly reduced when services are more readily available and more responsive to the realities of day-to-day life. Increased accessibility through appropriate hours of service, programs responsive to the needs of local residents, and increased provider understanding and respect for family and community life can encourage use of services and contribute to improved health status.

It is important to remember, however, that relocating services to the community does not immediately render them community *health* services. Many community-based services retain a medical focus on individual care and an illness orientation. If primary care services are provided, they are often individual-oriented rather than family-centered. They may occur according to prescribed medical protocols but may perhaps be limited to primary care, without concomitant population-based and clinical preventive care as described earlier. Although such care may address the immediate needs of one person or family, it may fail to fully promote and protect health. Knowledge of what else is happening in the community is essential in identifying risk to that person and to others who live there.

Environmental conditions conducive to health and community resources that complement or support health care are crucial. Without the full scope of effort ranging from care for individuals, to families, communities and entire populations, professionals cannot significantly improve society's health status. Only by examining aggregates can full appreciation for health and illness patterns and risks emerge, and for vulnerable populations to be identified. Population-focused care must serve as the basis of a health focused paradigm for care.

COLLABORATION: ENHANCING CAPACITY FOR COMMUNITY HEALTH CARE

There are a broad array of stakeholders in health care, including individuals and families in need of services; health professionals, health care organizations, and vendors that provide health care services and products; insurers, business and government that pay for care; and the broader community where the impact of poor health status is felt in reduced participation and productivity in day-to-day life.

Health care in and for the community requires careful consideration of people's lifestyles, issues of concern, and the availability or absence of resources to address them. All stakeholders need to be included. Only through this inclusionary process can understanding of key issues and perspectives occur, and only in this way can long-term significant changes be accomplished rather than simply short-term limited actions.

Partnerships of health care and multisector community organizations, working jointly instead of independently, are more likely to address many difficult issues, concerns, and needs related to health and the delivery of effective services to the community. They will be able to conduct a broad and comprehensive analysis of the issues and opportunities for health, and can contribute a wide array of resources to assist them in accomplishing the work of refocusing and implementing health care changes (Himmelman, 1992).

The term *collaboration* is used in many ways and has a variety of meanings to different people. A working definition is important to establish. Himmelman (1992) defines collaboration as "a voluntary strategic alliance of private and nonprofit organizations and groups to enhance each other's capacity to achieve a common purpose by sharing risks, responsibilities, resources, and rewards." Mattessich and Monsey of the Amherst H. Wilder Foundation (1992) similarly suggest that "collaboration is a mutually beneficial and well-defined relationship entered into by two or more organizations to achieve common goals. . . . The relationship includes a commitment to: a definition of mutual relationships and goals; a jointly developed structure and shared responsibility; mutual authority and accountability for success; and sharing of resources and rewards."

It is a higher level of involvement than simply cooperation or even coordination, although the term is often used interchangeably with these. Collaboration is a more durable and pervasive relationship that emerges as the participants develop mutual understanding, respect, and trust over time.

In a comprehensive review and analysis of articles in the professional literature regarding collaborative efforts, Mattessich and Monsey (1992) have identified a number of factors that influence the success of collaborations formed by human service and other organizations, including a supportive and facilitative environment, appropriate and inclusive membership, a structure and process for taking care of business, good communication, a shared vision and clear goals, and sufficient resources. Such efforts will require courage, patience, integrity, commitment, and a good dollop of humor as professionals establish relationships, envision health-oriented care, and undertake strategic interventions.

NURSING: REFOCUSING THE PROFESSION TOWARD HEALTH

This chapter emphasizes the importance of recognizing the challenges to nursing in a health-focused paradigm for care. Primary health care in the community requires careful consideration of the norms of practice. At all levels, nursing practice roles have been severely limited and controlled by the dominant medical ideology, which has restricted nursing's scope and medicalized health care, philosophy, education, and clinical practices (Watson, 1995). In this period of shifting the locus of the health care system, nursing must remain committed to its own human health and healing paradigm, and its roots in providing care in communities. At the same time, nursing must be willing to open itself to working in partnership with all participants in a primary health care model.

New practice settings, closer relationships with families within the context of their home and community life, partnerships with other health and social service providers, and relationships with community leaders and policy makers will form the foundation for practice in the future. Dr. Halfdan Mahler (1985), former director general of the World Health Organization, identified nurses as leading the way in primary health care. He predicted that the role of nurses would include moving from the medical/curing role in hospitals to primary health care in the community. This will "entail more innovation, greater responsibility and more involvement in program planning and legislation" (Anderson & McFarlane, 1996, p. 17).

Educators must reconsider nursing roles, responsibilities, and practice models for community-based and community-focused health care at all levels of professional preparation.

Frameworks for practice within these models must include an identified client (individual vs. aggregate), levels of responsibility, care setting, and levels of decision-making authority (Figure 1–6). Colleges

Figure 1–6
Levels of Education and Community Practice

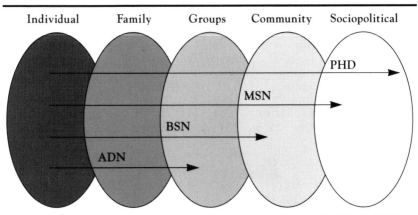

Individual   Family   Groups   Community   Sociopolitical

PHD

MSN

BSN

ADN

Note: Adapted from "Community as Client—A Multivariate Model for Analysis of Community and aggregate health risk" by S. Rogers, 1984, *Public Health Nursing, 1*(4), pp. 210–222. Reprinted by permission of Blackwell Science, Inc.

and universities have initiated a number of collaborative ventures to begin this process (Independence Foundation, 1995). The necessary knowledge for each level of practice is emerging, along with requisite competencies in direct care, communication, and management/leadership. At a 1996 meeting of the National League for Nursing practice councils, Lynn Rinke, Vice President of the Greater Philadelphia Visiting Nurses Association, noted that nurses will need to concentrate on *assessment, teaching,* and *management* of other personnel who will increasingly serve as direct caregivers. From these efforts will come improved standards for care, appropriate licensing and accreditation regulations, and health care financing policies and mechanisms for nurses.

CONCLUSION

As nurse educators, practitioners, and researchers move into this new health care paradigm, the profession must be willing to let go of old programs, methods, stereotypes, and myths associated with the illness-focused paradigm. Innovative, imaginative, and creative approaches to caring for the full range of clients across the care continuum must be devised. Osborne and Goebler (1993) note that a "let's make this work" approach by those who are unafraid to "dream the great dream" will provide the energy and commitment needed for this task. A willingness to take risks, to reward merit, and to celebrate successful initiatives in this area of professional development will richly benefit the community, the profession, and the health care system as a whole.

REFERENCES

Anderson, E., & McFarlane, J. (1996). *Community as partner.* Philadelphia: Lippincott-Raven.

Goeppinger, J. (1984). Primary health care: An answer to the dilemmas of community nursing. *Nursing Outlook, 1*(3), 129–140.

Green, L., & Kreuter, M. (1991). *Health promotion planning: An educational and environmental approach.* Mountain View, CA: Mayfield.

Himmelman, A. (1992). Local government and collaborative change. *Communities Working collaboratively for change.* Minneapolis: The Himmelman Consulting Group.

Independence Foundation. (1995). *Community-based health care initiatives.* Philadelphia: Annual Report.

Larson, E. (1995, July/August). New rules for the game: Interdisciplinary education for health professionals, *Nursing Outlook,* 23–27.

Mahler, H. (1985, October). Nurses lead the way. *New Zealand Nursing Journal.*

Mattessich, P., & Monsey, B. (1992). *Collaboration: What makes it work.* St. Paul, MN: Amherst H. Wilder Foundation.

Osborne, D., & Goebler, T. (1993). *Reinventing government.* New York: Dutton.

Rogers, S. (1984). Community as client—A multivariate model for analysis of community and aggregate health risk. *Public Health Nursing, 1*(4), 210–222.

U.S. Public Health Service. (1995). *Prevention report.* Washington, DC: U.S. Government Printing Office.

Watson, J. (1995). Advanced nursing practice and what might be. *Nursing and Health Care: Perspectives on Community, 16*(3), 78–83.

World Health Organization. (1978). *Report of the International Conference on Primary Health Care,* held in Alma Eta, USSR. Geneva, Switzerland: Author.

2

When Ambiguity Replaces Certainty

New Faculty Roles in Community Settings

M. Elaine Tagliareni
Susan Sherman

The process of leading a faculty group into new territory is more about not know-ing than knowing. The secret is in the searching for the answers, not in the answers themselves.

Waters, 1995, p. 75

Nursing leaders face a daunting task in today's uncertain and unpre-dictable world of health care. Compelled to develop interactive and con-temporary curriculum models without clear indicators to provide direction, faculty struggle to hold onto traditional approaches that are known and comfortable while voicing a desire to embrace change. They are troubled by broad goals that national organizations have established without furnishing prescriptions for action: Healthy People 2000 (U.S. Department of Health and Human Services, 1990); Nursing's Agenda for Health Care Reform (American Nurses Association, 1991); A Vi-sion for Nursing Education (National League for Nursing, 1993); the Pew Health Professions Commission (Shugars, O'Neil, & Bader, 1991). They search for right answers and yet, as Waters points out, the process of seeking new ways is more about not knowing than knowing. The need for faculty to find reward and fulfillment by being with students in emerging environments of care in ways that are presently unknown and untried is the most pressing and the most difficult challenge facing fac-ulty today. This was a lesson we learned well during our years as project principals in the W. K. Kellogg, Community College Nursing Home Partnership project, as we responded to the need for new faculty alliances and shifting curriculum paradigms. The many lessons learned during that project have influenced our thinking about the processes needed for change in and through nursing education today. It is these lessons that shape the ideas presented in this chapter.

CERTAINTY VERSUS AMBIGUITY: THE CHALLENGE TO FACULTY

As nurses, we are magnetically attracted to certainty. There are surely good explanations for our discomfort with ambiguity, both historical and sociological, but continuing to act as though there is always or almost always one right answer handicaps us now more than ever. (Waters, 1995, p. 75)

Coming to terms with ambiguity is not easy. It requires a posture that traditionally has not been played out in nursing education, where earnest desire to embrace innovation, has been contrasted by a tendency to retain traditional approaches that seem right because they are based on mental models of the past and because they are known and comfortable. But the old ways, developed when nursing educational levels had clearer boundaries and when acute care provided direction and focus to curriculum choices, no longer fully address the needs of the emerging, uncertain health care environment.

Today, professional education in the allied health sciences is concerned with balancing the known with the unknown. All health professions have been challenged to train tomorrow's practitioners for an uncertain future (Shugars, O'Neil, & Bader, 1991) that may require a variety of approaches, in diverse settings. Yet training for uncertainty has not been the historical posture of nurse educators. In fact, the concept of training used in nursing education for decades has traditionally referred to technical, objective-driven instruction primarily occurring in institutions. It is a valued and essential part of nursing education that includes skill acquisition, use of the nursing process, and knowledge of related physiological and psychosocial concepts. But this approach to nursing education, when not accompanied by other approaches, does not lend itself to interactive and collaborative learning (Bevis & Watson, 1989). It has not equipped students and faculty to accept ambiguity and to plan for it. It will not produce graduates to manage the fluid and rapidly changing work environment predicted for the future.

In her speech at the National League for Nursing biennial convention, Mary Catherine Bateson (1993) addressed the concept of ambiguity in the nursing profession. Bateson called for nurse educators to convey technical knowledge essential to safe nursing practice without making students rigid. She stated that throughout history, whenever changing trends or catastrophic events interrupt the status quo and create uncertainty and confusion, the natural tendency is to tighten control, to solve the problem of ambiguity with rigidity. In this age of health care reform, she challenged faculty to resist this temptation.

According to Bateson, the task for faculty is to develop a posture of "committed tentativeness" in graduates, to ground them solidly and firmly in the basics of professional practice and knowledge while fostering an environment that values creative thinking and actively encourages diverse approaches to care. To accomplish this outcome, faculty will need to make significant changes in current teaching learning strategies. For example, faculty need to spend less time in skills laboratory on fundamental topics such as bedmaking, simple dressings, and oral medications so that more time can be spent on delegation, teaching, and counseling skills needed in homes and community settings. If the emerging role of the nurse is one of management, assessment, and teaching, not direct provision of nursing care (as described in Section II), faculty will need to be less acute care focused. They will need to teach skills in relation to setting; for example, washing hands in the hospital, at the community-based day-care center, and in the home involves common principles, but when teaching hand-washing, faculty also must explore with students the subtleties of varied approaches in diverse environments of care. Committed tentativeness will demand that faculty ground students in the basics of nursing practice, including the nursing process, early in the nursing curriculum and then give up lecture time in later semesters to provide opportunities for students to think outside the box and develop personalized, creative care plans in collaboration with clients and families. It will require faculty to assist students to feel comfortable and competent with care planning that is firmly grounded in theory and practice standards but that changes based on personal meaning, context, and setting.

Committed tentativeness calls for "grounded improvisation" (Bateson, 1993). Like the jazz musician who practices eight hours a day to improvise in jazz concerts at night, the nursing student of tomorrow must experience a curriculum that quickly, intensively, and proficiently grounds them in the basics of theory and practice and then frees them up to think creatively, to experiment, to be innovative, to accept the ambiguous and highly personalized nature of health planning. Adherence to an institution-based curriculum, with a primary focus on diseases and their treatment, simply cannot accomplish this mandate. Students need meaningful exposure to new settings for practice that are "messy" (Shea, 1995, p. 42) and less clearly defined; they need to understand that textbook answers do not readily fit the health and illness experience for individuals and families in these settings; and most importantly, they need to find comfort and excitement in this realization.

WHY CHANGE IS SO DIFFICULT

Neither undergraduate nor graduate education in nursing or in education has prepared faculty for any but the behaviorist curriculum model . . . most faculty, regardless of academic degrees, have not been prepared for the shift in thinking and interacting with students (that is needed in nursing education today). (Bevis &
Watson, 1989, pp. 111–112)

One of the most common misconceptions about change is that change is viewed as an indication of failure. It is difficult for all individuals (and faculty are no exception) to move forward if they perceive that the impetus for change negates past successes. So often, faculty interpret the move to community-based, primary care models as a nullification of what was good and right about the acute care, disease-focused model. It is only natural that faculty, who were primarily educated as and hired because they were acute care specialists, would be conflicted about a move away from traditional approaches to curriculum design.

As Bevis and Watson (1989) suggest, faculty are not prepared to forsake institution-based curriculum strategies and shift to health promotion and disease prevention models of nursing care delivery. Nothing in the history of nursing has helped to ground faculty in a community-based health care system that requires a collaborative and colearner model of teaching and learning. Nursing faculty first learned to be nurses in a behavioral, content-laden, measurable, structured curriculum (Bevis & Watson, 1989). Objectives for learning flowed from an orientation to what to teach rather than how to teach. Teachers were traditionally aligned to content not to the process of learning. Nursing faculty's introduction to nursing and their allegiance to the profession occurred in a curriculum model where it was possible to learn "all" nursing content in the basic curriculum. And nursing faculty have taught subsequent generations of nurses using this same model, spending endless hours at curriculum planning meetings moving content from one semester to the other and debating the efficacy of adding or deleting content. In this context, there has been little time to think about the process of learning and to align the teacher with the student as the primary way to promote learning. Similarly, nursing faculty grew and developed as practitioners of nursing in an acute care, disease and hospital-based health care system. It is difficult, therefore, to think about health care in a system where the community is the focus of service delivery and to move from an allegiance to cure models of intervention to ones that include health promotion, disease prevention and health restoration. As faculty acknowledge the need to change education models to ones that are collaborative and interactive and to create community-based approaches to clinical learning, resistance and skepticism are a likely reaction.

THE NEED TO CELEBRATE THE PAST

The best way for faculty to move forward is to celebrate and feel good about past successes, about what they accomplished when the acute care hospital was the hub of the health care system, when traditional curriculum models based on specialties represented the norm, and when the expectations for nursing education and nursing practice were different. It is important for faculty to ask themselves both personally and collectively: What have been the most significant successes of our nursing curriculum? What value do we bring to nursing education? To our students? What shared values should we hold onto as we move forward? Addressing these questions and making a list of faculty responses to give all faculty and revisit periodically at faculty meetings is an essential first step in the change process. The key element in this process is for faculty to define past successes and to begin to recognize that those successes were measured within a different health care system, at a different place in history. In that context, decisions were right and competent and good. But past expectations can no longer define the future as it is becoming.

Moving forward requires creating a delicate balance between celebrating what has been done well and developing a sense of urgency based on the notion that what defined success in the past may, in fact, ensure the opposite in the future. Faculty must come to terms with the idea that some beliefs and assumptions that made them successful in the past will make them unsuccessful in a reformed health care system, especially if they define competency and value based on old expectations and skill sets. Demands to revise and adjust curriculum will mean those skill sets will change as competency is redefined and measured according to new expectations. It is the task of department heads and deans to help faculty not only to recognize past accomplishments but to celebrate them. At the same time, chairs and deans must provide opportunities for all faculty to free themselves from traditional approaches to curriculum design that cannot and will not hold true in future health care systems.

MENTAL MODELS OF CURRICULUM PLANNING

> *Mental models that act as barriers to change contain underlying assumptions that can't possibly hold true for the future. We must examine our mental models and discover the reality gap. Models unexamined remain unchanged. The inertia of firmly imbedded mental models can overwhelm even the best insights. (Senge, 1990, p. 176)*

Once faculty have celebrated a past filled with successes and have recognized that some of those successes will no longer define competence, they are ready to come face to face with their "sacred cows" or traditional mental models that have informed curriculum decisions in the past. This confrontation will allow faculty to challenge many untested assumptions and myths about curriculum planning.

> **Myth:** *Curriculum planning is synonymous with predicting the future.*

The only sure prediction for future events in health care is that nothing is certain. Much is happening already: hospital closings and mergers, changing demographics, the emergence of skilled care in the home and in nursing homes, increasing numbers of medically underserved in urban and rural environments. In this environment, curriculum development should be less about predicting future trends and more about planning for events that have already happened. Waiting for future events to unfold and to be clearly defined leads to exactly that, more waiting and subsequent inaction. One of the most effective faculty development strategies, learned during the Kellogg project, is to just start (Waters, 1991) and to accept what evolves, making adjustments and course corrections along the way. Faculty never made big mistakes, just minor missteps that created important learning opportunities.

Myth: *Curriculum planning must be sensible, practical, and realistic.*

Faculty are all too familiar with traditional approaches to the dreaded "major curriculum revision." Bevis and Watson (1989) refer to this process as "the 7-year itch," a time when faculty meet, and meet some more to debate issues such as integration, where to put what content, what to name the courses and whether or not to rework the program organizational framework (p. 113). The changes seem monumental to faculty and the energy and time required would indicate that strategic and substantial changes have occurred. It rarely has. This practical and sensible approach to curriculum planning is always safe. It involves making incremental, reactive changes to decreased hospital beds, increased patient acuity in institutional settings, and changing maternity and pediatric inpatient stays. We call it tinkering. In reality, it is not about planning strategically for a fundamental change in the focus of the nursing curriculum. It rarely leads faculty to a thorough examination of the direction of health care and the nurse's place in a reformed system; it does not produce a curriculum that trains and educates for uncertainty.

Throughout the years of the Kellogg project, a major dilemma for project faculty was whether the senior-level nursing home experience would dilute the learning program by taking students away from acute care. Faculty reasoned that students would not be as successful on the N-CLEX examination. It never happened. So too, during our last NLN accreditation visit, program evaluators were encouraged to visit and observe students in three pilot group experiences in community-based clinical settings. Faculty had developed clear outcomes (congruent with the program's organizing framework) that guided student learning in the pilot groups. Faculty alerted the evaluators that the outcomes were a work in progress and would change, no doubt, in subsequent semesters. The nursing program received full accreditation.

For us, developing curriculum strategies that are in transition or that represent a departure from usual norms is acceptable; in fact, it is preferable. The notion that curriculum planning needs to be guided by accreditation standards, N-CLEX norms, and graduate employment surveys is widely accepted by nursing faculty. We, too, adhere to these parameters but we try not to be constrained by them. We believe that taking risks usually works. With purposeful leadership and consistent support, faculty decisions are soundly based in teaching learning theory, and innovative clinical experiences are in concert with program philosophical beliefs. Trying to be certain takes time and energy; it is not necessarily time and energy well spent.

Myth: *The product of curriculum planning is more important than the process.*

Development of outcome criteria is the order of the day. Accreditation standards for academic departments as well as critical pathways in clinical settings call for compliance to qualitative and quantitative norms as measures of accountability. Outcomes are important. But the lessons learned along the way to outcome achievement are equally significant; in fact, they may play an even greater role in shaping program redirection.

During the Kellogg project, we discovered two very important notions about faculty movement toward curricular change. One, people change and forget to tell each other. Two, "faculty enlightenment comes not as an apocalypse, but as a slow dawn. You rarely see it happen . . ." (Waters, 1995, p. 82). We cannot overemphasize how important it is to provide opportunities for faculty to dialogue about lessons learned, to think out loud, to talk about the anxiety and fears that result from changes in the curriculum and to share achievements as well as disappointments. Faculty need to build on each other's experiences as they reframe and rethink program goals. Program outcomes need to be broad enough to encompass a wide variety of approaches. When outcomes present broad ends-in-view (Bevis & Watson, 1989) and are less prescriptive, an energetic and eager faculty will discover more diverse and creative strategies. This process is sometimes slow and often painful, but it will yield ideas and clinical learning opportunities that were not envisioned when outcomes were initially determined. Mueller and Henshaw (Chapter 12) provide a telling analysis of this process at Front Range Community College; their experience led to a reconceptualization of the nursing curriculum to include the full spectrum of health care delivery.

FACULTY TRANSITION TO
NEW PRACTICE SETTINGS

Task forces won't work unless the environment supports fluidity and informality; experimenting won't work if the context is wrong. Management has to be tolerant of leaky systems; it has to accept mistakes, support bootlegging, roll with unexpected changes, and encourage champions. (Peters & Waterman, 1982, p. 145)

The realization that faculty who take on new and experimental teaching assignments will suddenly feel like outsiders, and are often viewed by faculty peers as changing something valuable merely to be innovative and clever, is not new to us. Developing a senior-level nursing home placement at a time when acute care institutions were competing for nursing school graduates created ambivalence and uncertainty among faculty in the Kellogg project. Movement outside the comfort zone of traditional approaches to teaching in the acute care setting, coupled with a change in focus to rehabilitation and maintenance goals seemed illogical and untimely. The sense of unrest that developed both personally and collectively with both faculty and students clouded all curriculum decisions and influenced forward movement. But we survived and came to understand more fully that unrest and uncertainty during curriculum change are inevitable. Whether the curriculum change involves a major strategic restructuring (as at Broome Community College, Front Range Community College, and Northeastern University, described in Section IV) or a simple reallocation of course credits, faculty will long for the good old days. They will gravitate to comfort zones that reflect their own education and practice. The key to successful curriculum change is to expect this faculty response, to plan for it and to accept it. The winners in the curriculum reform movement will be those faculty groups who live with and seek out change, who thrive on broad, less prescriptive goals for action, who embrace ambiguity and who tolerate and welcome a state of flux and experimentation.

This is not a situation that nursing education leaders traditionally embrace. Chaos and paradox are in direct contrast to certainty and right answers. In our experience, the traditional approach to curriculum change is to try to help all faculty find comfort and ease during the change process. In the early days of the Kellogg project, we would discuss options for new clinical teaching methodologies by telling faculty how the changes would differ only slightly from previous approaches, hoping that a sense of continuity would prevent discord and apprehension. It never worked! Even mild tinkering leads to disruption in faculty harmony. Now we suggest a less compliant approach. Change is disruptive; it creates unavoidable uneasiness. Trying to prevent the inevitable robs faculty and department chairs of the energy needed for loftier pursuits.

Now we tell faculty and students that a new approach to curriculum, very often termed a "pilot project," will not be smooth and will entail use of untried and untested assumptions. But we also tell them that we will support them as pathfinders and we will provide formal mechanisms to debrief and receive encouragement. Then, we reward them for their vision.

According to a recent report of the PEW Higher Education Roundtable (1996), one of the key factors for successful faculty and department renewal is the leadership provided by a purposeful chair. The report stresses the importance of a chair who provides strong and decisive leadership, ". . . along with a spirit of teamwork and shared endeavor among department's membership. A chair must embody the spirit of camaraderie and collegial exchange that makes possible the achievement of common goals within the department. . . . To be effective, a chair must establish the tone and context for department discussions of the curriculum, making certain that teaching and learning are principal subjects of discourse" (pp. 9–10). It is impossible to exaggerate the need for deans and curriculum chairpersons to provide an environment that supports and rewards faculty in the change process.

At the Nursing Leadership Conference in Orlando, Florida (1995), Dr. Venner Farley introduced us to the 30-70 rule for faculty change. According to Farley, 30 percent of the faculty constitutes a critical mass for effective curriculum change. The remaining 70 percent will follow slowly or perhaps not at all, but it is a waste of time to seek 100 percent faculty compliance before initiating "pilot" experiences. During the Kellogg project, we conducted a survey asking over one hundred project faculty to describe their biggest fear about curriculum revision. To a person, they identified the "faculty at home who do not want to change." We now know that these project faculty were the critical 30 percent. With adequate support from a purposeful chair in the form of frequent meetings to discuss progress and receive a fresh perspective on unfolding events, as well as the selection of strong and flexible students to participate in the initial pilot groups, faculty will be empowered to develop effective strategies to initiate strategic curriculum change. Strong

leadership and a work environment that supports and fosters experimentation will overcome the inevitable uncertainty and ambivalence.
Change will be incremental, not dramatic, but innovation will unfold.

CHANGES IN THE FACULTY TEACHING ROLE: BECOMING AN EXPERT NOVICE

Students are not the only novices; any nurse entering a clinical setting where she
or he has no experience with the patient population may be limited to the novice level
of performance if the goals and tools of patient care are unfamiliar. (Benner, 1984,
p. 21)

Movement to new practice settings is never easy for nursing faculty.
Strategies for practice and teaching do not transfer intact from one
setting to another. Early in the Kellogg project, we developed a model to
describe faculty transition to the nursing home setting (Waters, 1993,
pp. 29–32). A major assumption inherent in model development is that
for faculty to fully understand the environment of a new practice setting
and take on new teacher roles, they must first become novices in that
setting. Yet faculty are not complete novices in a new setting. They
bring expert knowledge of teaching-learning strategies to that setting
and convey years of experience from acute care on curriculum decisions.
Assuming the novice posture presumes that these characteristics will not
transfer intact and that faculty will be open to experiences in new settings, in order to learn new and different ways of knowing students and
clients. We coined the term "expert novice" to describe the posture
needed to fully assimilate the unique characteristics of a new practice
setting:

Being an expert novice then means being open to the differences in the practice
setting in order to recognize opportunities for innovative nursing approaches to health
care delivery. It means entering a new practice setting, knowing that previous acute
care models cannot be wholly transferred to the new setting. (Tagliareni & Murray,
1995, p. 367)

Over the years, we have explored components of the faculty transition
model with our colleagues nationally. This process has led to the development of a model that compares the teaching role in the acute care setting, described as "One Way," with teaching approaches required in

community-based settings (which are derived from lessons learned in the nursing home) described as the "New Way" (Figure 2–1). We have refined the model to provide direction and clarity for faculty considering movement to community settings.

The faculty teaching role identified as the new way encompasses a proactive, interactive approach to teaching, where learning is collegial, and students and faculty are colearners in new practice environments. Traditional methodologies commonly used in acute care are described as reactive, for example, the activity of instructors as they respond nonstop to dry IVs, numerous discharges, and frequent requests for pain medication. In the "One Way" model, the clinical day is spent reacting to rapid changes in the environment. A successful day is often measured by the number of skills performed by students. In this model, the instructor and the student engage in parallel play and work alongside hospital nursing staff (Tagliareni, Sherman, Waters, & Mengel, 1991). Although students and staff discuss treatment options and immediate concerns about changes in patient status, opportunities for mutual care planning are often limited.

In the community, as well as in the nursing home, the required shift from reactive to proactive teaching and from parallel play to interactive caregiving is both threatening and unsettling to faculty. Because it is different, it just does not seem "right." In the community, faculty must create the learning opportunities as there is often very little to react to. In the community, it becomes essential for both faculty and students to collaborate with interdisciplinary staff and with families to understand significant health care needs. The interventions take time to listen, to collaborate, and to plan health care outcomes together. This change in focus can seem ineffective and less than rewarding. It is not; it is merely

Figure 2–1
Faculty Teaching Role

One Way	New Way
Reactive	Proactive
Parallel play	Interactive play
Value goals that cure or assist dying	Value goals that maintain and promote optimal functional ability with individuals/families
Learning: Teacher controlled	Learning: Collaborative, collegial, colearner

different. But it does require that department and curriculum chairs allow faculty time to use trial and error in developing new clinical experiences. It directs chairs to support all faculty during their adjustment to a proactive and collaborative teaching and practice environment.

Through years of experience with senior-level nursing students in the nursing home, we learned to value nursing goals that assist residents to function optimally in their own safe and familiar environment and to define wellness according to the resident's perspective. These approaches reflect the unique practice patterns in the nursing home. In previous writings, we have told the students' stories about personal caregiving within the high-tech, rapid-pace technological world of present-day health care (Tagliareni, Mengel, & Sherman, 1993; Tagliareni, 1993). Now, we are struck by the similarities in practice patterns found in the nursing home and in community-based settings. In both settings, the focus of care is on personalized care planning to maximize potential and improve the living environment. Refining previous work that contrasted the practice patterns in acute care, a transition setting, with the practice patterns in homelike settings, such as the nursing home (Tagliareni, Mengel, & Sherman, 1993), we submit a model (Figure 2–2) that describes the differences between the parallel worlds of acute care and community nursing practice. We believe it is essential to consider these differences when teaching in community settings and to value goals related not only to cure and dying well but also to appreciate and teach care-planning activities directed toward maintenance and promotion of optimal functional ability for patients and families. This approach requires faculty to reframe and recast content on common health problems, as well as redesign approaches to care planning in the clinical environment. For example, when teaching the topic of congestive heart failure, it is essential to incorporate concepts related to how individuals live with heart failure in the community, how they cope with functional deficits, how progress is measured during the rehabilitative period, as well as to discuss nursing responses to acute exacerbation of symptoms.

Years of teaching one way, whether in acute care at the bedside or in less structured settings, requires that faculty move out of their comfort zones and embrace new approaches to teaching. The old way will not work in a consumer-driven, primary care health care system and it will not assist faculty and students to personalize nursing care for clients and families. A fundamental change in the faculty teaching role is, we feel, the better way in new community-based environments of care.

Figure 2–2
A Model to Understand the Work of Nurses in
Acute Care and Community-Based Settings

Acute Care Setting	Community-Based Setting
Specialized care planning focusing on a crisis event. Interventions are standardized and sporadic.	Comprehensive care planning within the context of current and past life events. Interventions are personalized and continuous.
Goals relate to resolution of acute, identified problems using technology and efficiency.	Goals relate to assisting individuals and families to function optimally in a safe and familiar environment.
Rewards derive from making connections with patients and families in the context of helping them to get better or die well.	Rewards derive from knowing individuals and families over time, maximizing potential, and improving the quality of the living environment.

A successful core of nursing practice occurs when the nurse exercises the choice and the self-confidence to merge the knowledge and the values learned in both settings into a personal practice paradigm.

The Future Involves More Searching

The discovery by Waters (1995) that the key to faculty development and curriculum reform is found in the searching for answers, not in the answers themselves, may seem in sharp contrast to some of the ideas presented in this chapter. At times, we spoke about what faculty must do and described essential curriculum concepts and teaching roles. It is not our intent to prescribe approaches to curriculum revision or to suggest that certain practices must necessarily be included in community-based experiences. Those choices will evolve as each faculty group makes decisions that fit their own students and their own unique communities. There is no magic formula for curriculum reform; no one design will fit all nursing programs uniformly. Neither rigidity nor standardized, homogenized approaches to teaching and learning will solve the problem of an ambiguous, uncertain health care future. Redefinition will come from faculty creativity and innovation; the future is up to us.

REFERENCES

American Nurses Association. (1991). *Nursing's agenda for health care reform*. Kansas City, MO: Author.

Bateson, M. C. (1993, June). Speech presented at the biennial convention of the National League for Nursing, Boston, MA.

Benner, P. (1984). *From novice to expert*. Menlo Park, CA: Addison-Wesley.

Bevis, E. (1993). All in all, it was a pretty good funeral. *Journal of Nursing Education, 32*(3), 101–105.

Bevis, E., & Watson, J. (1989). *Toward a caring curriculum: A new pedagogy for nursing*. New York: National League for Nursing Press.

Farley, V. (1995). Speech presented at the Nursing Leadership Conference, Orlando, Fla.

National League for Nursing (1993). *A vision for nursing education*. New York: Author.

Peters, T., & Waterman, R. (1982). *In search of excellence*. New York: Harper & Row.

Pew Higher Education Roundtable. (1996, February). *Policy perspectives* (pp. 1–12). Philadelphia: Institute for Research on Higher Education.

Senge, P. (1990). *The fifth discipline: The art and practice of the learning organization*. New York: Doubleday Currency.

Shea, C. (1995). In P.S. Matteson, (Ed.), *Teaching nursing in the neighborhoods*. New York: Springer.

Shugars, D., O'Neil, E., & Bader, J. (1991). *Healthy America: Practitioners for 2005, An agenda for U.S. health professional schools*. Durham, NC: Pew Health Professions Commission.

Tagliareni, E., Sherman, S., Waters, V., & Mengel, A. (1991). Participatory clinical education: Reconceptualizing the clinical learning environment. *Nursing and Health Care, 12*(5), 248–263.

Tagliareni, E. (1993). The nursing home clinical: New horizons for capitalizing on a caring experience. In Burke & Sherman (Eds.), *Gerontological nursing: Issues and opportunities for the twenty-first century* (pp. 37–43). New York: National League for Nursing Press.

Tagliareni, E., Mengel, A., & Sherman, S. (1993). Parallel worlds of nursing practice. In Burke & Sherman (Eds.), *Ways of knowing and caring for older adults* (pp. 91–105). New York: National League for Nursing Press.

Tagliareni, E., & Murray, J. (1995). Community focused experiences in the ADN curriculum. *Journal of Nursing Education, 43*(8), 366–371.

U.S. Department of Health and Human Services, Public Health Service. (1990). *Healthy people 2000: National health promotion disease prevention objectives*. Washington, DC: Department of Health and Human Services Publication 91-50212.

Waters, V. (Ed.). (1991). *Teaching gerontology*. New York: National League for Nursing Press.

Waters, V. (1995). *The narrative enlarging*. New York: National League for Nursing Press.

3

When Community Becomes More Than a Place

New Curriculum Choices in Community Settings

M. Elaine Tagliareni
Susan Sherman

The call for nursing faculty to reexamine their collective beliefs about nursing education and nursing practice in light of health care reform is old news. For over a decade, all levels of nursing leadership have called for curriculum reform that would address the complex and personalized work of nursing. To become "faculty of the community" (Moccia, 1993, p. 474) requires altering a curriculum orientation that is almost entirely based on the practice of nursing in hospitals. Yet, nursing education has remained traditional and static with an acute care focus that continues to direct both its process and content. Although nurse educators have verbalized an understanding of and a commitment to new models of health care delivery, the move to revolutionize nursing practice and nursing education and to make important adjustments in teaching-learning paradigms is slow and cumbersome. This chapter will look briefly at this phenomenon as well as provide ideas for reframing traditional thinking about both community and a community-based curriculum.

UNDERLYING ASSUMPTIONS AND MENTAL MODELS

In Chapter 2 we discussed the need for faculty to discard sacred cows, or myths about curriculum planning. This notion also applies to beliefs about clinical learning.

35

Tagliareni and Murray (1995) provide four assumptions or mental models that have been revered as truth in ADN education. They suggest that challenging each of the following assumptions will offer opportunities for new ways to think about nursing education and nursing practice:

1. *Community nursing* is a universal term that has common meaning to nurse educators.
2. The focus of associate degree nursing education is on the individual client at the bedside in the hospital setting.
3. Concepts about nursing in community settings and management skills should be taught at the end of the program of study (simple to complex).
4. The nursing process is the primary tool to teach and practice nursing.

Bevis and Watson (1989) write about several untested assumptions that have assumed the power of axioms for nursing faculty. These include:

1. Everything the student may ever need to know (and should know) must be covered in the curriculum.
2. Given the same assignments and environment, students will have much the same experiences and learn much the same things.
3. Every student needs to have as nearly as possible the same experience as every other student.

And finally, in our discussions of mental models with faculty across the country, additional sacred cows have consistently emerged. These include:

1. The best learning takes place when the instructor is present.
2. Faculty can control the learning environment.
3. For the past 40 years (advent of ADN programs), "community" has been the only clear-cut subject area difference between associate and baccalaureate curricula.
4. ADN graduates practice in structured settings and BSN graduates practice in less structured settings.

Although the specific sacred cows may vary among faculty groups, the need to come to terms with them is paramount. These beliefs do not represent unsound thinking. They make sense in an educational system that is acute care based and behaviorally oriented. They provide the foundation for nursing curricula that have been effective and come from a proud historical tradition. Now, though, they are outdated. Faculty need to challenge these mental models and free themselves to move toward new definitions of community and new approaches to collaborative, interactive models of teaching.

COMMUNITY AS PLACE, APPROACH, AND STATE OF MIND

Many nurses are coming to home health assuming that they will employ the same set of skills and knowledge base as in their acute care practice. No assumption could be more naive. (Stulginsky 1993a, p. 403)

For nursing faculty reared in traditional curriculum models over the past 40 years, community describes a place where nursing takes place in homes and community health agencies, outside the walls of the hospital and the nursing home. The traditional approach to nursing education reserves community for BSN clinical experience and eventual graduate employment. This mental model needs changing. Community, we maintain, is more than a place and more than home care. In a reformed health care system focused on health promotion and disease prevention, it is an approach to curriculum design. Community is a state of mind.

In the definition of community as place, the assumption is that home care is the pivotal teaching environment for community-based clinical experiences. This assumption derives from faculty's basic preparation in public health nursing, when as student nurses, faculty managed a caseload of clients for visiting nurse associations or city health departments. This model, still utilized in many BSN programs, is at best, too little and too late in the socialization process needed to make a difference in how students accept and integrate community health practices (Matteson, 1995). As associate degree nursing faculty look to embrace community-based learning experiences, they too often gravitate, automatically, to home health care agencies. Faculty traditionally teach what they know and what they have known for over a lifetime of practice.

There is no doubt that home care is growing at a phenomenal rate. The U.S. Commerce Department considers home care one of the fastest growing segments in the medical market (Weinstein, 1993). Estimates indicate that as many as 9 to 11 million Americans need home care services, representing an annual growth rate of 12 percent from 1991 to 1994 (National Association for Home Care, 1994). Certainly, care of individuals and families in the client's place of residence is rapidly becoming the preferred recovery environment paid for by managed care insurance companies. It is also true that high-tech home therapy is on the rise as well as hospice care. All these trends contribute to make home care an attractive placement for clinical learning. But to define community nursing as synonymous with home health care alone is to negate the opportunities for health promotion and disease prevention activities carried out in senior centers, schools, churches, day-care centers, homeless shelters, nursing centers, and other community-based agencies (U.S. Department of Health and Human Services, 1990). Sections IV and V in this book describe approaches to community-based care that include new and innovative models for home health care preparation as well as methodologies for developing educational partnerships with other community settings where, often, no other kinds of health care services are available. This book is designed to broaden the definition of community as place, and to offer a wide range of alternatives for clinical placement. It is time for faculty to explore neighborhood-based programs that augment a community-based approach to curriculum design, instead of limiting themselves to traditional placements.

This move requires that faculty embrace community focused thinking. In the past, faculty have been traditionally institution focused. An allegiance to the hospital and to hospital-directed approaches to skills laboratory and content delivery has characterized nursing programs for decades. Skills are taught from the context of the hospital environment, and care planning related to chronic management of health problems is often overlooked, or barely talked about. Theory presentations in the classroom most commonly focus on acute management of a common health problem and long-term management at home or in community settings is often an afterthought, taught in the last 5 to 10 minutes of class, if at all. Discharge planning is overtly proclaimed by faculty to be an integral part of current nursing practice, but when time is short, the subject is often sacrificed for "one more nursing diagnosis." This methodology to curriculum implementation comes from faculty's comfort with traditional approaches that are historically institution based.

Community-focused thinking requires faculty to create clinical schedules that account for a variety of settings at different times throughout the day. It presumes that students will not be guaranteed a predetermined clinical lab each semester and that they will acknowledge the benefits of this approach. It suggests that the traditional clinical group of 10 to 1 is no longer viable and that, new methodologies to monitor students in smaller groups at two or three agencies should be the norm. And finally, it necessitates that theory presentation in the classroom incorporate planning and evaluation of both health maintenance and health restoration goals, including individuals' and families' adjustment to the recovery process. Being community-focused requires faculty to transform their thinking away from institutions and to continually and consistently ask themselves if decisions made at faculty meetings about course and clinical requirements reflect a community orientation. The acute care, institutional approach served nursing and nursing education well for decades; its viability in a community-based health care system now needs to be questioned.

Our concept of community as a state of mind is an outgrowth of the empirical research conducted by Joanne Rader in the nursing home setting. Rader (1993) sought to determine appropriate interventions to prevent agitation and restlessness in individuals with cognitive impairment who wander. She writes, "When I accompanied several residents and their spouses to the home they had left to come to the nursing home, they requested to go 'home' in that environment also. I sensed that they were seeking not so much a geographic place as a state of mind" (p. 46). According to Rader, these individuals were not looking to be back in a physical space, but to capture the sense of purposefulness and security associated with people and situations that had previously made the person feel most connected and comfortable.

Community is not just a geographic place; it is also a mind-set: It represents a total redirection for nursing faculty. Their resistance and skepticism represent a need to go back "home" to an institution-based environment that previously brought feelings of safety and belonging. But the future requires that nursing faculty focus the nursing curriculum on health and primary health care delivery, as well as on health restoration, and assign a significant and meaningful part of the student's basic education to settings outside the hospital and the nursing home. Community as a state of mind necessitates the full integration of community concepts throughout the program of learning; content about community cannot be relegated to one course in the final semester. Concepts about collaborative models, maintenance of functional ability during recovery, and rehabilitation in noninstitutional settings must become a jumping-off point for all classroom discussions and for the development of new clinical partnerships. There is no going home to old ways, only opportunities to rediscover the sense of competency and connectedness in a restructured and reformed health care system.

TRADITIONAL AND COMMUNITY-BASED SETTINGS

The mistake we nursing educators made and continue to make is to try to use one paradigm to answer all our needs. (Bevis, 1993, p. 103)

As a result of research conducted during the Community College Nursing Home Partnership project, a model was developed that described the nature of nurses' work in acute care and long-term care settings (Tagliareni, Mengel, & Sherman, 1993). The impetus for development of this model was the tendency of project faculty to replicate conventional approaches to clinical teaching in the acute care setting when developing collaborative relationships with nursing homes. On reflection, we theorized that the two settings reflect different institutional values and ethics and that the work in each setting would vary. Building on that earlier work, we are presently suggesting a model that represents the unique practice patterns in traditional (institution) and community settings. This model (Figure 3–1) provides direction for student learning objectives and helps faculty acknowledge differences between settings and select teaching methodologies accordingly.

The traditional setting for nursing practice, the hospital, is structured with clear protocols for delivery of nursing services. The high-stimulus, short-stay environment is focused on the individual patient. Nursing interventions are directed toward resolution of a crisis situation or an acute exacerbation of a long-term chronic illness. Although this is a "transitional setting, not a landing place for cure" (Tagliareni, 1993, p. 32), nursing actions are primarily cure oriented and outcomes are determined according to standard protocols or critical pathways. The nursing process is the principal methodology for teaching problem-solving and for evaluating patient outcomes. The acute care setting is a world characterized by "standardized treatment protocols, high acuity and shortened length

Figure 3–1

Traditional Settings	Community-Based Settings
Focus	**Focus**
Structured	Borrowed
Individual	Individuals/Families within their environment
Cure	Optimal function
Technology where skills are standardized	Technology where skills are adapted
Outcomes	**Outcomes**
Standardized	Personalized
Methodology	**Methodology**
Nursing process	Mutual problem solving

of stay" (Tagliareni, Mengel, & Sherman, 1993). This world presents a striking contrast to the community-based environment.

Stulginsky (1993a, 1993b) refers to the community setting as borrowed, where control belongs to the clients in their home. Borrowed settings rapidly shift nursing's power base and require collaboration. The collaborative model brings mutual problem-solving to determine shared needs and shared responsibility for health care delivery expanding the focus of care to the family. "The family is the primary context in which health promoting activities occur and therefore potentially the most immediate source of health-related support and education for the individual" (U.S. Department of Health and Human Services, 1990, p. 85). Families live in neighborhoods and health care is delivered close to where they live, work, rest, and pray. This is a completely different context from the structured settings of institutions and requires culturally sensitive approaches to management of health problems. Given this perspective, we reasoned that students should begin the program of learning with a general orientation to the family rather than to the individual nurse-patient relationship. Even in the acute care setting, the focus on family makes sense and fosters a more comprehensive approach to planning for rapid discharge.

The primary goal of care in community settings is to improve the ability of individuals and families to function in a safe and familiar environment. This may involve cure methodologies, but it also encompasses a commitment to maintenance and health promotion goals. Perhaps the curriculum implication for faculty is assisting students to value well-being and improved functional performance as highly as they regard resolution of an acute illness. Both nursing actions are an integral part of nursing practice; both deserve emphasis in a fully integrated community-based curriculum. Flexibility and creativity are essential components of the nurse's role in providing highly skilled care. "There is no common baseline from home to home" (Stulginsky, 1993b, p. 478). The intimacy that comes from knowing individuals and families in their own homes and neighborhoods implies familiarity and a sense of personalization not always experienced in the short-stay, high stimulus hospital setting. Helping students to understand and appreciate the fine differences between maintaining distance and establishing trust and rapport in a professional, healing relationship is a powerful and essential part of learning to be a nurse in community environments. The context-based outcomes are influenced by past history and cultural and socioeconomic factors as well as personal agendas.

> *Neighborhood learning experiences help students understand that health care is an integral part of everyday life, that health care is not a service done to or for someone else nor the prerogative of one group of professionals. They learn from their interactions that health is a personal value and individual responsibility based on cultural and family norms. (Matteson, 1995, p. 96)*

Learning this important lesson helps the student define nursing and nursing interventions as less predictable than hospital and institution-based outcomes.

Throughout the years of the Kellogg-sponsored Community College Nursing Home Partnership project, we questioned the use of the nursing process as nursing's primary teaching tool (Waters, 1991). The neat, behaviorist approach to solving problems does not support personalized and collaborative thinking. We now ask, how can we develop models of critical thinking that foster participatory problem-solving, that help students to pay attention to context and appreciate individuals and families as part of a larger neighborhood community? Creative problem-solving includes opportunities to reflect, learn through discovery, and challenge assumptions about values and belief systems. These components must be part of a community learning experience so that students begin to truly understand and appreciate personalized, neighborhood-based care. Sections IV and V of this book provide numerous examples of innovative approaches as nursing faculty experiment with collaborative, interdisciplinary experiences in the community that foster critical thinking.

Addressing the complementary yet different practice patterns of traditional and community-based settings offers an approach to rethink nursing practice and assign new meaning to nursing education in a reformed health care system. Both environments play an integral role in this new system—one is not better than the other. Consideration of the traditional and community based model, described earlier, may help nursing educators ease the transition and provide direction for student learning outcomes in both settings.

TEACHING STRATEGIES IN A COMMUNITY-BASED CURRICULUM

Proactive and interactive teaching that emphasizes promotion of optimal functional ability within the client/family's familiar and safe environment requires a fresh approach to curriculum design. Throughout this book, and especially in Sections IV and V, national faculty describe projects that incorporate many of these concepts. This chapter includes a synopsis of essential components (Figure 3–2) in a community-based curriculum to assist faculty in identifying critical reform strategies.

Community Involvement throughout the Program of Learning

Since we believe that community is an approach to curriculum planning as well as a state of mind, it follows that community-based experiences

Figure 3–2
The Essential C's of a Community-Based Nursing Curriculum

Community involvement throughout the program of learning.

Collaborative models of teaching and learning in all nursing courses.

Critical thinking for culturally sensitive care delivery.

Care planning over time in selected clinical environments.

need to be integrated throughout the program. These experiences are not limited to clinical time in community settings. At Community College of Philadelphia we utilize seminar time to receive feedback from students after they have conducted interviews with well-elders in the community (Waters, 1991, pp. 71–72), with women experiencing pregnancy, and with families who have a member with a chronic disability. Students participate in health fairs and screening activities in every course. Classroom time includes case studies of individuals in the community who are coping with multiple chronic health problems. Section IV describes nursing programs at Broome Community College, Northeastern University, and Front Range Community College that have included the full spectrum of health care delivery in all nursing courses.

Collaborative Models of Teaching and Learning in All Nursing Courses

The traditional leveling of nursing programs (simple to complex) usually involves movement from a focus on the individual to the family and to the community. In this approach, strong emphasis is placed on the one-to-one relationship between nurse and client and most learning experiences for students include the development of care plans written in isolation, usually after the clinical day. Management principles for groups of clients are often taught late in the total curriculum, after students master care planning with individual clients. In a community-based health care system, faculty need to rethink these concepts of curriculum progression (Tagliareni & Murray, 1995).

Future nursing practice demands a nurse who understands collaborative practice (Shugars, O'Neil, & Bader, 1991), who can negotiate mutually derived health care options and who shares the task of providing health care with other disciplines and with neighborhood agencies. These competencies demand a curriculum that initially incorporates concepts about community and, more specifically, experiences in collaborative caregiving. Assigning beginning students to work in teams to develop beginning care plans and to complete patient care assignments is helpful. Later experiences can include group in-service teaching assignments, group presentations at staff planning conferences and clinical opportunities to interact with both agency personnel and community residents to develop mutually derived health promotion activities. In a community-based model, the focus is redirected to collaborative practice, away from individual assignments and care planning.

Critical Thinking for Culturally Sensitive Care Delivery

Problem-solving or the nursing process is a framework for solving problems; it may not have critical thinking as an element. (Bevis, 1993, p. 104)

Throughout the Kellogg project, we wrestled with nursing education's love affair with the nursing process (Waters, 1991; Tagliareni & Murray, 1995). In a health care environment where both faculty and students are asked to accept ambiguity and develop personalized care plans based on context, traditional approaches do not always fit. Certainly the nursing process, as a standardized, universally accepted approach to developing a strategy for nursing action, provides a fundamental knowledge base for beginning nursing students. But, it falls short as the only methodology for care planning because its behaviorist, linear framework impedes collaborative decision making and creative, personalized approaches.

Critical thinking involves reflection, the challenging of assumptions, understanding of a reality context, and discovery learning. It can only be learned in a collaborative, colearner relationship with faculty. Critical thinking cannot simply be read about or taught solely in the classroom. Essential teaching/learning strategies include experiences in community environments where students and faculty challenge beliefs about traditional health care practices, about how and why clients and families access care, about what factors define adherence to treatment protocols—and where students and faculty discover and plan together creative approaches to culturally competent nursing care. The pilot projects described in this book are based on components of critical thinking. These projects speak to efforts by innovative faculty to support students to be flexible, critical thinkers in a world of health care that, at present, is ambiguous and uncertain.

Care Planning over Time in Selected Clinical Environments

One of the most startling discoveries made during the Kellogg project was that, prior to the initiation of project activities, a majority of students had never cared for a client over a two-week period. The rapid turnover in acute care, together with the belief, adhered to by faculty, that clinical learning is enhanced by a change in client care assignments on a weekly basis, contributed to this phenomenon. As project faculty moved to the nursing home with groups of senior-level nursing students who cared for the same 8 to 10 residents over five to six weeks, they realized that knowing residents over an extended period contributed to personalized care planning and facilitated students' ability to evaluate progress and adapt nursing actions to the living environment. Students had time to challenge assumptions, use reflection as an effective thinking tool and collaborate with peers and staff to assign personal meaning to care plan decisions. All these competencies are essential to community-based nursing practice. We know that the short-stay, high-tech, high-stimulus acute care environment does not lend itself to reflective practice. Experiences in acute care are essential to provide a foundation for safe and effective nursing practice. But knowing clients in personal environments of care and knowing them over time are also essential components to clinical teaching practices in a reformed nursing curriculum.

DEVELOPMENT OF A NEW VISION

As nurse educators fully embrace innovative and revisionary frameworks for curriculum design in a community-based health care system, every nursing faculty group needs to define a vision for action. As reported by the Pew Higher Education Roundtable (1996), "Few departments systematically sought the feedback of all the constituencies they served—and none could be said to understand that, regardless of individual performance, the group succeeded or failed as a whole" (p. 5). It is imperative that nursing departments design ways to develop faculty commitment to a collective vision that calls for a greater sense of teamwork, a curriculum that is futuristic and responsive to changing health care agendas and promotes an environment where risk taking and creative approaches to curriculum planning are respected and supported. Only then will nursing faculty recast, revitalize, and restructure for the future.

REFERENCES

Bevis, E. (1993). All in all, it was a pretty good funeral. *Journal of Nursing Education*, 32(3), 101–105.

Bevis, E., & Watson, J. (1989). *Toward a caring curriculum: A new pedagogy for nursing.* New York: National League for Nursing Press.

Matteson, P. S. (1995). *Teaching nursing in the neighborhoods.* New York: Springer.

Moccia, P. (1993). Nursing education in the public trust: A faculty of the community: No unreal loyalties for us. *Nursing and Health & Care, 14*(9), 472–474.

National Association for Home Care. (1994). Basic statistics about home care, 1994. Washington, DC: Author.

Pew Higher Education Roundtable. (1996, February). *Policy perspectives.* Philadelphia: Institute for Research on Higher Education. 1–12.

Rader, J. (1993). Empirical trial and error: Learning from practice. In Burke & Sherman (Eds.), *Ways of knowing and caring for older adults* (pp. 43–49). New York: National League for Nursing Press.

Shugars, D., O'Neil, E., & Bader, J. (1991). *Healthy America: Practitioners for 2005, an agenda for U.S. health professional schools.* Durham, NC: Pew Health Professions Commission.

Stulginsky, M. N. (1993a). Nurse's home-health experience—Part I: The practice setting. *Nursing & Health Care, 14*(8), 402–407.

Stulginsky, M. N. (1993b). Nurse's home-health experience—Part II: The unique demands of home visits. *Nursing & Health Care, 14*(9), 476–485.

Tagliareni, E. (1993). Issues and recommendations for associate degree education in gerontological nursing. In Heine (Ed.), *Determining the future of gerontological nursing education* (p. 32). New York: National League for Nursing Press.

Tagliareni, E., Mengel, A., & Sherman, S. (1993). Parallel worlds of nursing practice. In Burke & Sherman (Eds.), *Ways of knowing and caring for older adults* (pp. 91–105). New York: National League for Nursing Press.

Tagliareni, E., & Murray, J. (1995). Community focused experiences in the ADN curriculum. *Journal of Nursing Education, 43*(8), 366–371.

U.S. Department of Health and Human Services, Public Health Service. (1990). *Healthy people 2000: National health promotion disease prevention objectives.* Washington, DC: Department of Health and Human Services Publication 91-50212.

Waters, V. (Ed.). (1991). *Teaching gerontology.* New York: National League for Nursing Press.

Weinstein, S. (1993). A coordinated approach to home infusion care. *Home Healthcare Nurse, 11*(1), 15–20.

SECTION II

Competencies for Future Practice

4

Nursing Competencies in Community Settings

Results of a Community-Based DACUM Activity

M. Elaine Tagliareni
Andrea Mengel

In the fall of 1994, nursing faculty at Community College of Philadelphia recognized the need to reexamine the nurse's role in a community-based health care system. The faculty assumed that in a community-focused curriculum the knowledge for effective nursing practice would differ from traditional approaches. Experience from the nursing department's eight-year involvement in the W. K. Kellogg Community College Nursing Home Partnership project taught faculty that movement away from a totally acute care curriculum focus changed both the teaching-learning paradigms and the settings where graduates seek initial employment.

A method used in the W. K. Kellogg project for formulating competency statements in new settings of practice was the "Developing a Curriculum" (DACUM) process, which was designed to assist expert practitioners to identify essential competencies for safe and effective practice in their field. In essence, the expert practitioners inform curriculum decisions by suggesting a path for faculty to follow. In the Kellogg project, the competency statements based on current practice in nursing homes became the foundation on which to build curriculum models (Tagliareni, 1991).

Because this methodology had proved so successful in the past, faculty sought funding to initiate a DACUM of nursing practice in community-based settings. The project, funded by the Independence Foundation of Philadelphia, identified four objectives:

1. Identify 12 to 15 community health nurses to participate in the DACUM process.

2. Generate a list of competencies through the DACUM process describing current and future practice in community-based settings.

3. Convene an expert panel of community health nurses to analyze the DACUM competencies in light of future practice initiatives and public policy.

4. Develop new curriculum models for integration of the identified community-based practice competencies that are appropriate to associate degree nursing graduates.

THE DACUM PROCESS

In June 1995, 14 nurses from settings outside acute and long-term care met in Philadelphia. The DACUM participants represented both urban and rural settings and a variety of practice environments outside institutional settings: ambulatory care, HMO practices (6 participants); home health nursing (3 participants); Visiting Nurse Association (3 participants); nurse managed home health agencies with a focus on maternal child health (2 participants). The DACUM participants represented 2 to 14 years of experience in community settings, with an average of 5 years.

The techniques used to conduct the analysis involved brainstorming and consensus. Participants began their work by listing, from their individual experiences, the categories into which they believed their work could be classified. Once all the categories were named to the satisfaction of all the participants, the group listed all the skill areas that constitute the nurse's role within a category. At the conclusion of the 1½-day process, participants prioritized the categories and the skills into a list of competency statements (Figure 4–1, on pages 54–57). Discussion among the participants focused on the three highest priority categories: assessment, coordination of care (management), and teaching. Although these categories are commonly used to describe current nursing practice, participants acknowledged that additional skills expand traditional definitions of assessing, managing, and teaching, and broaden essential practice competencies. These skills include providing access to health care, ensuring eligibility to services, referring to appropriate community resources, and facilitating interdisciplinary plans of care. Additionally, participants speculated that categories describing Promotion of Personal Safety (K), Facilitation of Reimbursement (M) and Marketing of Services (N) identified a skill base for nurses that may, in fact, belong specifically to nursing practice outside acute and long-term care settings. The challenge for the nursing faculty was to incorporate both sets of skills in basic nurse preparation, within the framework of Community College of Philadelphia's integrated curriculum.

EXPERT PANEL

An expert panel of community health nurse educators and advanced practice community health nurses ($n = 6$) convened to analyze the DACUM results considering forecasts for future practice and the goal to integrate DACUM competencies into the nursing curriculum. Members of the panel were surprised that communication was not identified as a separate category of practice, especially since communication skills are an integral part of community nurse practice. It was noted, however, that communication skills are well detailed within each practice category of the DACUM competencies. Panel members also wondered why primary health care was not addressed in the DACUM categories. Perhaps provision of primary health care services by nurses "at the front line" is a futuristic practice arena that is not currently played out in the health care environment.

Panel members, together with the project evaluation consultant, encouraged the faculty to utilize the DACUM competencies to plan learning experiences in community-based settings for associate degree nursing students. Faculty and students had already completed an initial community assessment of the college's immediate neighborhood, the 19130 zip code, and determined that a variety of learning experiences in diverse settings were available for student placement (Chapter 17). The problem faculty faced was determining which learning experiences in the community were essential. Through discussion and brainstorming, faculty asked the following question to guide evaluation activities and curriculum development: What makes a learning experience essential to the role of the associate degree nursing student as defined by the

Figure 4–1
Community College of Philadelphia Department of Nursing
DACUM Analysis of Nursing Practice in Community Settings

Conduct Initial and Ongoing Assessment	A1. Anticipate barriers to access to care.	A2. Identify life-threatening emergencies.	A3. Determine eligibility for services.	A4. Refer to appropriate agencies based on eligibility.	A5. Review patient record: discharge orders, pre- and posthospital medications and treatments, primary physicians.	A6. Assess home safety and environment (using all senses).	A7. Conduct physical assessment (all systems).
Coordinate Care	B1. Evaluate needs for coordinated services.	B2. Coordinate care with payer as appropriate.	B3. Advocate for patient.	B4. Set realistic short- and long-term goals involving patient and family.	B5. Adapt care to culture.	B6. Interact with patient and family throughout care.	B7. Communicate with physicians verbally and in writing.
Teach Patients, Caregivers, Staff	C1. Promote patient rights and responsibilities.	C2. Provide instruction to patient and caregiver regarding access to health care providers.	C3. Assess knowledge and literacy level.	C4. Prioritize teaching needs.	C5. Set goals.	C6. Identify willing caregiver.	C7. Develop individualized teaching plans.
Provide Skilled Nursing Care in a Community-Based Environment	D1. Maintain patient dignity.	D2. Provide care in a nonjudgmental manner.	D3. Adapt infection control techniques to home care and outpatient settings.	D4. Identify strategies to adapt patient care principles to home environment.	D5. Provide psychosocial support.	D6. Provide terminal care.	D7. Conduct health tests and screening tests.
Promote Restorative Care	E1. Promote skin integrity.	E2. Assist with ADLs.	E3. Perform ROM.	E4. Position patients.	E5. Manage incontinence.	E6. Ambulate and transfer patients.	E7. Maintain orthopedic devices.
Manage Medication Therapy	F1. Administer medications safely.	F2. Manage IV therapy.	F3. Administer SQs, IMs and intradermal.	F4. Manage pain.	F5. Adapt the medication regime to patient needs.	F6. Store and transport medications approximately.	F7. Check expiration dates.

* Boxed items represent those competencies best taught in community settings.

8	9	10	11	12	13	14	15
A8. Assess pain and wounds.	A9. Assess nutritional status and dietary compliance.	A10. Perform psychosocial assessment to include cultural, economic, sexual and role.	A11. Conduct functional and activity tolerance assessment.	A12. Conduct family assessment (support system).	A13. Identify community resources available (including church, clubs, etc.).	A14. Determine patient motivation and compliance.	A15. Develop a care plan.
B8. Maintain communication with all other disciplines and community resources.	B9. Facilitate interdisciplinary plan of care.	B10. Participate in interdisciplinary case conferences.	B11. Adopt plan of care to time and reimbursement constraints.	B12. Identify and access community resources.	B13. Maintain accountability for patient care.	B14. Purchase services, equipment.	B15. Supervise ancillary personnel.
C8. Adapt teaching to the patient/caregiver abilities.	C9. Utilize a variety of creative teaching tools to improve compliance and understanding.	C10. Provide written material.	C11. Adapt teaching to home/community environment.	C12. Evaluate teaching.	C13. Maintain a patient medical file on site.	C14. Instruct staff regarding patient care.	
D8. Perform venipuncture for laboratory tests.	D9. Perform KGs.						
E8. Operate speciality equipment (i.e., beds, hyperbaric chambers).							
F8. Develop a system for medication administration (color code, pill-box etc.)	F9. Assess patient compliance with medication.	F10. Supervise ancillary personnel giving medication.	F11. Obtain prescriptions as necessary.	F12. Identify cost-effective suppliers of medications.	F13. Contact physician regarding alternate medications according to patient finances.	F14. Correlate medical diagnosis with medications.	F15. Dispose of contaminated materials and sharps (OSHA).

Figure 4–1 (Continued)

	1	2	3	4	5	6	7
Perform Treatments	G1. Maintain patient airways.	G2. Care for patients with tracheotomies and ventilators.	G3. Perform wound care.	G4. Care for ostomies.	G5. Insert and care for tubing and catheters.	G6. Provide prenatal care.	G7. Perform postpartum care.
Maintain Documentation	H1. Obtain consents and advanced directives.	H2. Record patient problems and actions taken.	H3. Document progress related to care plan.	H4. Chart all communication (phone calls, visits, teaching services).	H5. Notate medications.	H6. Record follow-up activities and lab tests/reports.	H7. Initiate photos or diagrams of wounds.
Solve Problems	I1. Listen actively.	I2. Consult with peers, supervisors, and other health care providers.	I3. Follow formal/informal chain of command.	I4. Conduct research.	I5. Collect data for identified research studies.	I6. Evaluate new products.	I7. Participate in quality assurance activities.
Develop Organizational Skills	J1. Organize a work area.	J2. Prioritize assigned responsibilities.	J3. Reassess schedule according to changes.	J4. Maintain flexibility regarding schedule.	J5. Read maps.	J6. Maintain updated and current resource list.	J7. Plan ahead.
Promote Personal Safety	K1. Assess the address/neighborhood for safety, crime, physical structure.	K2. Schedule visits according to patient preference and personal safety.	K3. Coordinate the visit with other providers.	K4. Identify unsafe situations.	K5. Maintain contact with your office, as necessary.	K6. Plan for safety when transporting equipment.	K7. Store equipment and supplies out of site.
Demonstrate Professionalism	L1. Practice within the scope of the nurse practice act.	L2. Maintain licensure and insurance.	L3. Adhere to policy/procedures of agency.	L4. Follow OSHA guidelines.	L5. Renew CPR certification.	L6. Obtain specialty certifications.	L7. Continue education.
Facilitate Reimbursement	M1. Discuss reimbursement methods.	M2. Identify criteria for reimbursement.	M3. Verify eligibility of patient for reimbursement.	M4. Explain insurance benefits to patient.	M5. Obtain proper address for insurance.	M6. Negotiate for reimbursement.	M7. Monitor changes in benefit/supply reimbursement.
Market Services	N1. Conduct community needs assessment.	N2. Identify services.	N3. Provide services as marketed.	N4. Identify agency and contact phone number and address, to patient and family.	N5. Participate in community health fairs.	N6. Develop community networks.	N7. Support community-related projects.

8	9	10	11	12	13	14	15
G8. Provide newborn care.	G9. Apply hot and cold packs.	G10. Feed patients with disabilities.	G11. Perform tube feedings.				
H8. Document discharge planning treatment options.	H9. Use a problem-oriented approach.	H10. Sign or initial all documentation.	H11. Chart concisely, legibly, timely, and objectively.	H12. Use medical terms and abbreviations appropriately.	H13. Maintain confidentiality.	H14. Identify requirements for record storage.	H15. Utilize computer for documentation.
I8. Read and critique literature.	I9. Apply current research to patient care.	I10. Suggest changes to procedures to improve flow of care.					
J8. Utilize available resources.	J9. Develop a system for documentation.	J10. Maintain and organize equipment and supplies.	J11. Revise daily plan based on outcomes.	J12. Demonstrate assertiveness skills.	J13. Manage time effectively.	J14. Keep records for tax purposes.	
K8. Lock facility when alone.	K9. Adhere to universal precautions.	K10. Seek assistance in dealing with threatening situations.	K11. Follow established emergency procedures.	K12. Utilize good body mechanics.			
L8. Participate in professional organizations.	L9. Adhere to professional standards adapting to environment.	L10. Identify current legal and ethical issues.	L11. Demonstrate professional behavior/attitude.	L12. Allow patient freedom of choice to select agency, MD, services.	L13. Complete incident reports.		
M8. Adapt documentation to insurance guidelines.	M9. Complete reimbursement required forms.						
N8. Market agency to insurance company.	N9. Initiate appropriate referrals.						

DACUM process and by experiential learning? Three criteria were established to consider a learning experience essential:

1. The learning experience contributes to the development or mastery of competencies that are identified as unique to the practice of community nursing as determined by the DACUM analysis.
2. The learning experience contributes to the development or mastery of competencies that the faculty identify to be "best taught" in the community.
3. The learning experience contributes to the development or mastery of competencies determined by the faculty to be essential to meet the nursing needs in the local (19130 zip code) community.

BEST-TAUGHT COMPETENCIES

The concept of "best taught" competencies emerged during the Kellogg project. Faculty participants assumed that while all DACUM competencies were essential to providing nursing care to older adults, some competencies were specific to nursing care of frail older adults with multiple chronic health problems and that the nursing home setting provided a special opportunity for mastery of select competencies. These competencies became the foundation for clinical objectives in the second-level nursing home experience.

Nursing faculty reasoned that a similar analysis of the community-based DACUM competencies would provide direction for learning objectives in community settings. Faculty assumed that many skills described in the DACUM were universal to all of nursing practice and that only some skills represent practice specific to community settings. Therefore, a cohort of nurses from acute care and long-term care were asked to evaluate the community DACUM competencies in relation to practice in institutional settings. Those competencies determined to be essential by 90 percent or more of the cohort group are listed in Table 4–1 and describe core competencies for nursing practice in all three settings: acute care, long-term care, and community settings. Faculty were amazed with the consistency of responses; nurses from acute care and long-term care consistently eliminated certain competencies in 11 of the 14 categories. Those competencies not considered

Table 4-1
Core Competencies for Acute Care, Long-Term Care
and Community Settings

A. Conduct Initial and Ongoing Assessment
    7. Conduct physical assessment (all systems).
    8. Assess pain and wounds.
    9. Assess nutritional and dietary compliance.
    10. Perform psychosocial assessment to include cultural, economic, sexual role.
    11. Conduct functional and activity tolerance assessment.
    12. Conduct family assessment (support system).
    14. Determine patient motivation and compliance.
    15. Develop a care plan.

B. Coordinate Care
    3. Advocate for patient.
    4. Set realistic short- and long-term goals involving patient and family.
    6. Interact with patient and family throughout care.
    8. Maintain communication with all other disciplines and community resources.
    9. Facilitate interdisciplinary plan of care.
    13. Maintain accountability for patient care.

C. Teach Patients, Caregivers, and Staff
    1. Promote patient rights and responsibilities.
    4. Prioritize teaching needs.
    5. Set goals.
    7. Develop individualized teaching plans.
    8. Adapt teaching to the patient/caregiver abilities.
    14. Instruct staff regarding patient care.

E. Promote Restorative Care
    1. Promote skin integrity.
    2. Assist with ADLs.
    3. Perform ROM.
    4. Position patients.
    5. Manage incontinence.
    6. Ambulate and transfer patients.
    7. Maintain orthopedic devices.

F. Manage Medication Therapy
    1. Administer medications safely.
    2. Manage IV therapy.
    3. Administer SQs, IMs and interdermal.
    4. Manage pain.
    5. Adapt the medication regime to patient needs.
    7. Check expiration dates.
    9. Assess patient compliance with medication.
    15. Dispose of contaminated materials and sharps (OSHA).

Table 4–1 (*Continued*)

G. Perform Treatments
   1. Maintain patient airways.
   2. Care for patients with tracheotomies and ventilators.
   3. Perform wound care.
   4. Care for ostomies.
   5. Insert and care for tubing and catheters.
   9. Apply hot and cold packs.
   10. Feed patients with disabilities.
   11. Perform tube feedings.

H. Maintain Documentation
   2. Record patient problems and actions taken.
   3. Document progress related to care plan.
   4. Chart all communication (phone calls, visits, teaching services).
   5. Notate medications.
   6. Record follow-up activities and lab tests/reports.
   7. Initiate photos or diagrams of wounds.
   9. Use a problem-oriented approach.
   10. Sign or initial all documents.
   11. Chart concisely, legibly, timely, and objectively.
   12. Use medical terms and abbreviations appropriately.
   13. Maintain confidentiality.

I. Solve Problems
   1. Listen actively.
   2. Consult with peers, supervisors, and other health care providers.
   3. Follow formal/informal chain of command.
   4. Conduct research.
   10. Suggest changes to procedures to improve flow of care.

J. Develop Organizational Skills
   1. Organize work area.
   2. Prioritize assigned responsibilities.
   3. Reassess schedule according to changes.
   4. Maintain flexibility regarding schedule.
   7. Plan ahead.
   8. Utilize available resources.
   12. Demonstrate assertiveness skills.
   13. Manage time effectively.

K. Promote Personal Safety
   9. Adhere to universal precautions.
   12. Utilize good body mechanics.

Table 4–1 (*Continued*)

L. Demonstrate Professionalism
 1. Practice within the scope of the nurse practice act.
 2. Maintain licensure and insurance.
 3. Adhere to policy/procedures of agency.
 4. Follow OSHA guidelines.
 5. Renew CPR certification.
 7. Continue education.
 9. Adhere to professional standards adapting to the environment.
 10. Identify current ethical and legal issues.
 11. Demonstrate professional behavior/attitude.
 13. Complete incident reports.

descriptive of practice in institutional settings may, in fact, be more indicative of skills that are unique to nursing practice in community settings and are determined to be competencies best taught in community settings. Those competencies best taught in community-based experiences are illustrated as boxed competencies in Figure 4–1.

IMPLICATIONS FOR CURRICULUM

Following a series of focus groups with the cohort group to validate survey results and assist faculty to more fully understand the rationale for selection of core competencies, nursing faculty at Community College of Philadelphia met in groups to discuss the best taught competencies and to plan learning experiences around pivotal issues that emerged from the DACUM analysis.

Access to Care

The issue of referral to appropriate agencies and identification of community resources emerged as an essential skill for community nurses. Faculty have developed experiences in all four semesters to help students to understand that acute care is a transitional environment, that recovery occurs outside the hospital and that without knowledge of community agencies and the skill to facilitate coordination with those agencies, nursing care is incomplete and discharge planning is inadequate. In the first nursing course, students conduct an assessment of their own neigh-borhood, identifying agencies where health and human services needs are met for local residents (Chapter 17). In the second semester, students present a seminar describing the purpose of one of the agencies discov-ered in the previous semester and discuss how that agency facilitates adaptation to chronic illness. In the third semester, students conduct a series of interviews with a family that utilizes community agencies to maintain and promote the health of one of its members who has a long-term, chronic illness. In the final semester, students practice in select community agencies in the college neighborhood. Throughout all four semesters, students plan discharge for clients in the acute care setting. It is expected that students will utilize inter-disciplinary personnel to de-termine eligibility for referral services and teach clients about the neces-sity of accessing care to prevent complications and promote health. This area of curriculum redesign directly corresponds to the best taught com-petencies related to referral of services and reimbursement for care.

Adaptation of Nursing Skills

The DACUM best taught competencies require that faculty adapt nurs-ing skills to emerging environments of care. Rather than add more con-tent related to skill acquisition, the DACUM assisted faculty to refocus existing skill content, especially in the areas of medication manage-ment, assessment, documentation, and teaching-learning evaluation methods. One faculty member commented, "All the examples I give in class are hospital based. The students asked me about nasogastric intu-bation in the home setting and, once again, I realized how critical it is for me to broaden my perspective and include examples outside of acute care." In Sections IV and V, national faculty discuss methodologies for adapting skills to home care and other community settings. Addition-ally, new skill development, such as health fairs and community assess-ment, are considered.

Safety

Once practice moves out of the institutional setting, the issue of per-sonal safety becomes paramount. As students conduct interviews in clients' homes, actively participate in community needs assessment activities, and deliver nursing services in community agencies, faculty are cognizant of the need to teach safety tips and to assist students in identifying unsafe situations. Faculty consulted with local police and campus security officials to plan for student safety and instructed students to travel in small groups during community assessment experiences. Other safety measures are still evolving as faculty and students implement safety strategies during experiential learning activities.

Market Services

As health care moves from an altruistic to a competitive, economic model, nurses must learn to wisely balance the economic model with a caring orientation. Helping individuals and families understand what services nurses provide and teaching them how to access those services is clearly indicated as a best taught competency, a skill critical to current nursing practice. Students at Community College of Philadelphia participate in health fairs throughout all four semesters and conduct community needs assessments in both first- and second-year courses. Not only do they learn about health promotion and disease prevention initiatives, but they interact with individuals outside the institutional setting, teaching them about their health and well-being and broadening the public's understanding of the services that nursing offers outside traditional settings. Students learn to sell themselves and their profession; they are empowered in the process. Although this outcome of community health fairs and community assessment activities was unanticipated, faculty now realize that these experiences are a practical and timely way to begin to teach marketing of nursing services and to expose students to delivery of these services in less structured environments. This outcome of community-based learning has become one of the most compelling lessons learned by both students and faculty.

Future Plans

The faculty intends to conduct further research to analyze the DACUM competencies and to further develop curriculum models based on the DACUM skills. Refinement and updating of essential competencies for safe and effective future practice for associate degree nursing graduates will emerge through continued faculty discussions, experiential learning in community settings and dialogue with practicing nurses throughout the full spectrum of health care delivery settings.

REFERENCES

Tagliareni, E. (1991). What and how of student learning activities. In V. Waters, (Ed.), *Teaching gerontology* (pp. 65–91). New York: National League for Nursing Press.

5

Nursing Competencies in a Rural Setting

Linda L. Vance
Susan C. Youtz
Bonnie L. Ashcroft

The clinical placement of nursing students in a rural nursing center has particular merit when considering the juxtaposition of today's managed care environment and the critical need for health services in rural areas. In 1995, the National Governors' Association observed that although rural residents comprise approximately one-quarter of the U.S. population, they do not have the same level of access to basic primary health care services that is available to other Americans.

Health care delivery in rural communities is complicated by poverty, inadequate transportation, geographic distance, an aging population base, alcohol and drug abuse, and rural economic decline. There is a critical need to improve access to health care services while simultaneously controlling health care costs (Tyman & Orloff, 1995). This chapter is presented with special attention to the parallel developments of reduced health care dollars, expansion of managed care, and increasing need for primary health services in rural areas.

Local and regional governments and states are all interested in identifying mechanisms to ensure that rural residents have access to cost-effective primary and preventive health care services. Recognizing the serious concerns associated with access to health care services in rural central Pennsylvania, the Philadelphia-based Independence Foundation provided The Pennsylvania State University School of Nursing with a seed grant in 1993 to study the establishment of rural nursing centers. This planning grant allowed School of Nursing faculty to expand an existing commitment to infuse rural health content

65

throughout undergraduate and graduate curricula, while examining ways to provide meaningful community-based clinical experiences in a rural nursing center.

In 1994 the School of Nursing, in collaboration with the Home Nursing Agency of Altoona, received funding from the Independence Foundation to establish two rural nursing centers in central Pennsylvania. Since that time, activities have been directed toward implementing all aspects of center operation including the provision of services, planning for student experiences and faculty practice, and evaluating all elements of center operation.

In this chapter, multiple contexts and perspectives are presented that provide the framework for the implementation of community-based clinical experiences in a rural nursing center. Two overarching themes are the importance of access to health care services for rural residents and the impact of managed care on the current health care environment.

The richness of practical experience for the student in a rural nursing center site depends, in part, on clearly defining the context in which learning is to occur. The two components addressed in this chapter are the dynamics of the managed care environment and the unique experiences that can be achieved in the rural community.

MANAGED CARE ENVIRONMENT

Health care at the turn of the century will be defined by models of practice that are emerging as a result of the need to reduce costs while providing a broader continuum of care. Although many believe that "hospitals will remain the cornerstone of health care service" (Porter-O'Grady, 1994), the challenges and opportunities for nurses working in community settings will be greatly expanded. "New clinical and managerial roles will likely be created by the spread of capitation (payment of a preset fee for specific medical interventions). . . . it is in the economic interest of capitated providers to keep people out of costly treatment facilities" (Buerhaus, 1996, p. 7). Further, Barger (1991) identified increasing opportunities for nurses in the managed care environment.

In theory, capitation and managed care promised to bring about managed competition and yield reduced costs; however, the paucity of services in rural areas prohibits that development. The documented shortage of providers in rural communities (Barnett & Bigbee, 1991; Stratton, Dunkin, & Juhl, 1995) will require quite different service delivery management than is anticipated in urban environments. Yawn (1994) points out that "because the population numbers are inadequate to support competing networks, the providers are required to collaborate to lower costs" (p. 11).

Instead of managed competition, these authors note that managed collaboration will be the successful model. Practice opportunities in a rural nursing center will provide both faculty and students with the competencies and skills necessary to be a leader in multidisciplinary collaboration.

RURAL CONTEXTS

The unique opportunities available for nurses in rural areas result from the intrinsic nature of the people, resources, and structures of their communities. As indicated earlier, health care resources in the rural community are limited both in numbers and levels of education and expertise. For example, in 1988 nearly 70 percent of all U.S. hospital closings occurred in rural areas (Kagawa-Singer, Pelusi, & Underwood, 1995). In Pennsylvania alone, nearly half of the rural counties rely exclusively on small hospitals or have no hospital at all (Pennsylvania Office of Rural Health News, 1994).

Recruitment and retention of health professionals, especially in light of reduced health care funding, continues to be difficult in rural communities. "Although about 25 percent of the population lives in rural areas, only 13 percent of all patient care physicians practice there. Only 17 percent of the nation's nurses live in rural areas and one in seven of these actually works in the city" (Kagawa-Singer, et al., 1995, p. 8). Bigbee (1993) notes that the "ratios of RNs per 100,000 population in 1988 for the United States as a whole was 675 but was 385 in counties with less than 50,000 population" (p. 135). Bigbee (1993) also states that rural nurses have lower educational levels than their urban counterparts. Other researchers have also identified the limited number of nurses in rural communities. Stratton, et al. (1995) support the idea that, while the controversy may continue regarding the existence of a nursing shortage, there is little disagreement about the lack of nurses in rural areas.

Limited health care for rural residents has many causes. In addition to an insufficient number of providers, the economy of rural communities compounds the issue of access to care. Demographic studies of rural areas indicate that there are higher numbers of elderly in rural communities as well as greater numbers of children living in poverty (Kagawa-Singer et al., 1995). *The State of the Child in Pennsylvania* (Richmond & Steketee, 1995) states that during the 1980s the rate of children in poverty increased in rural areas 24.4 percent compared with 7.1 percent in urban centers. Few dispute that children and elderly are often those populations at greatest risk and most in need of accessing health care services.

Family structure and employment also affect the rural economy. Rural family incomes are often dependent on unskilled jobs connected with farming, mining, logging, or truck driving. Many are self-employed or work for small companies where health insurance is limited or nonexistent. Lee (1993) also noted that rural people are not inclined to consider health matters routinely and, thus, utilize health care services less than their urban counterparts. Further, the limited population base often does not support the establishment of large health care facilities and multiple providers.

Rural culture is often not conducive to the recruitment of health care professionals. Many note the lack of collegial interaction, little access to continuing professional education, and limited personal and professional resources—all of which have the potential to hamper the recruitment and retention of nurses in rural areas. Further, a nurse who is the product of an urban educational emphasis may, for a variety of reasons, feel uncomfortable in a rural setting. The cosmopolitan culture and highly technical delivery of health care services in a fast-paced urban environment offers numerous opportunities for specialization. Opportunities for networking and peer interaction are readily available, whereas in rural settings there is greater opportunity for health care providers to practice using a generalist approach in an environment that values independence and autonomy.

CLINICAL EDUCATION FOR NURSES IN RURAL SETTINGS

Limiting nurses' education to an urban setting may restrict the nurse's experience of health care delivery to a single perspective. Bandman and Bandman (1995) argue for the importance of nurses being educated "to identify and analyze health care issues from the perspective of more than one point of view" (p. 5). Exposure to varied cultures, including the rural culture, provides that opportunity. The lack of exposure and opportunity to experience a rural community limits a nurse's comfort zone to the urban environment, thus decreasing the likelihood of a nurse ever practicing in a rural setting.

Further, an urban nurse who is comfortable in multifaceted urban neighborhoods may feel awkward within the often homogeneous farming, mining, or single-industry community. Feelings of cultural and geographic isolation combined with a need for enhanced professional opportunities often will deter nurses from moving to or remaining in a rural community.

There is no question that many factors contribute to the unequal deployment of nurses in rural settings referred to by Stratton et al. (1995). However, the same factors that are part of the problem can also create opportunities. Bushy (1992) contends that interdisciplinary collaboration will be required to overcome limited rural resources. Successful health care outcomes will depend on the cooperative interaction of a wide variety of community leaders and health care providers who represent different disciplines and multiple levels of education. The independence that many rural nurses experience in their practice may in fact foster the interdependence that is associated with collaboration. Barnett and Bigbee (1991) note that nurses are well suited to provide leadership in this collaboration because they are "fundamentally educated as generalists" (p. 168). A rural nursing center as a locus of practice will enable both faculty and students to gain important new collaborative experiences in the rural health care arena.

The success of rural health promotion will depend in large measure on the relationships that are developed with both local residents and community leaders. Rural residents know their communities best and their acceptance often dictates the success of innovative health care programs. Marczynski-Music (1994) states that one of the significant guiding principles relating to community health is that "health actions be made *with* people and not *to* people, and that the people have input and participation in health planning" (p. 167). She believes a paradigm shift is underway and that local communities may lead the way in transforming the vision of health care delivery.

Nurses can play a significant role among rural populations if they understand rural attitudes and values about work, health, the importance of friends and family, and the utilization of resources. Lenz and Edwards (1992) attributed part of the success of their nurse-managed primary care center in rural eastern Tennessee to the recognition that the residents were the "experts" on their own community and that both problems and assets belonged to them. Early student involvement in grassroots activity and in developing community partnerships provides the foundation for using local resources throughout a student's entire nursing career.

In addition to providing opportunities to become acculturated and understand the dynamics of rural communities, rural nursing centers encourage concentrated, nurturing relationships between students and their preceptors. Because of the shortage of rural health care providers, students often feel more integral to the activities in the nursing centers. The pace of rural interaction also permits the preceptor time to teach, demonstrate, and build a relationship that fosters meaningful mentoring. Corrigan (1992) describes the development of preceptorships in rural Arizona. Students made the following observations about their preceptors:

> *She was never too busy to give assistance or information or listen . . . [I was] very much [a part of the staff]. The primary nurses were frequently in touch with me, asking questions, and referring to my charting, reviewing concerns, and progress of clients. . . . We planned experiences together to coordinate with client families, but work was completed independently. (p. 347)*

Rural nursing centers permit the development of satisfying preceptorships in addition to demonstrating to students the value of *all* relationships.

The remainder of this chapter focuses on several philosophical perspectives and competencies needed to enable the nurse to play a pivotal role in the delivery of health services to rural communities. A rural nursing center provides a unique location for practice that can place the nurse as central to the client, the physician's practice, the tertiary or primary hospital, the community, and other health and human service providers. Successfully influencing individual and community health outcomes not only requires a broad perspective regarding the scope of nursing practice, but also necessitates an understanding and appreciation of the entire health and human service delivery system and the environment that surrounds the consumer.

PHILOSOPHICAL PERSPECTIVE

One of the first considerations to address when students enter the rural nursing center setting is their philosophy about health and human services and their attitude about rural residents. The traditional acute care paradigm of nursing care is often determined and at times constrained by the clinical expertise needed in a specific work area. Clinical skills set nurses apart from other disciplines and often from each other. Further, in the acute care setting, nurses receive and implement the physician's orders, specific to the presenting problem. Time, financial and human resources, and other institutional restrictions often limit further involvement with the client, as well as other professionals who may play a significant role in the health outcomes of the client and his or her family.

Clinical practice in a rural setting often requires a completely different approach. To be a significant participant in affecting the health outcomes of individuals and families in rural communities, the nurse must have a broader view of the community and its residents. For example, where a hospital setting may have a physical therapy department, a rural community often considers itself fortunate to obtain the services of a visiting physical therapist once every two weeks. A physical therapy assistant or a nurse may be the primary person responsible for an individual's therapy. Further, due to time constraints and the size and geographic spread of the nurse's caseload, a family member or friend may need to be a significant member of the care team.

The hospital social service department may have a totally different look in a rural community. Instead of three or four people available at a specific hospital extension number, the community may have a school guidance counselor, a local minister, a child welfare worker, and a housing authority representative, all of whom provide part of the social service function.

The successful nurse will value each colleague for that person's skills and competencies and will recognize that successful health outcomes often hinge on multidisciplinary communication and collaboration. In the rural setting, duplication often refers to the number of calls or coordinating activities that must take place for a person to receive services—not to the services themselves.

Another important philosophical perspective in the rural area involves consumers. As each acute care setting has a culture that influences how nurses will perform their services, so, too, does each community. Often, the scarcity of available services, the rural culture of independence, and the insider/outsider paradigm inherent in rural communities may combine to limit consumer utilization of services. Limited utilization causes many an inexperienced consumer to lack the skills needed to access the appropriate service when it does become necessary. The vocabulary of the health care professional is, in itself, daunting to laypersons—particularly those who are removed from major health centers by distance and interest.

While understanding the politically conservative, traditionalist nature of the rural resident, it is also important to value other features of rural residents and their community structures. To be successful, the nurse needs to involve residents in the development of any services to be offered. Further, any involvement of rural community residents will require the demonstration of a demeanor that is respectful of the rural residents' way of life and values.

THE RURAL NURSING CENTER
PRACTICE SETTING

The rural nursing centers described in this chapter are located in rural central Pennsylvania. The sites are part of the Rural Nursing Centers Project, a collaborative initiative established by The Pennsylvania State University School of Nursing and the Home Nursing Agency with funding from the Independence Foundation of Philadelphia. Nursing students have been integrally involved with the project since the earliest phases of project implementation.

The nursing centers were established in rural communities whose census profiles and geographic distance from physician practices and hospitals indicate they are medically underserved locations. The central region of Pennsylvania is predominantly rural, often isolated from easy access to health care services by mountainous terrain. The beauty of the Appalachian Mountains, the quiet country roads, and widespread family farms often hide poverty level incomes and unemployment rates higher than the statewide rate (U.S. Census, 1990).

While some counties in central Pennsylvania have small cities that classify them as metropolitan, most areas are rural and have documented need for comprehensive primary health care services. Many central Pennsylvania communities have been designated as Health Professional Shortage Areas (HPSAs) or Medically Underserved Areas (MUAs) by the U.S. Department of Health and Human Services (1992). One rural nursing center is located in southern Huntingdon County, which has been identified as a county-at-risk, characterized by residents who have significant medical need with limited access to health care facilities. Another nursing center is located in a small tightly-knit blue-collar community of less than 700 people who must travel 15 miles to obtain health care. Nearly 20 percent of the residents are elderly and the poverty level is 50 percent higher than the state average.

Penn State School of Nursing and the Home Nursing Agency, a large multicounty, multiservice Visiting Nurses' Association, combined their expertise to establish and operate the nursing centers. The project is governed by an advisory board composed of community representatives and equal representation from the School of Nursing and Home Nursing Agency. The goals of the project are:

1. Rural underserved residents will have access to high-quality, primary and preventive services.
2. Clinical experiences in rural communities and with families will prepare Penn State University undergraduate, graduate, and practitioner nursing students for service in underserved rural communities.
3. The innovative partnership model (Penn State University/Home Nursing Agency) for Nursing Centers will become part of the mainstream in the health care continuum and provide a model for other communities.
4. Through collaborative involvement of Penn State University faculty and the Home Nursing Agency professional staff, opportunities for research and development will lead to interdisciplinary approaches that meet the health and human service needs of rural residents.
5. The activities of this project will be evaluated according to established outcomes developed by the Nursing Center Board.
6. If appropriate, a process for replicating the model in other locations will be developed.

Penn State School of Nursing faculty and students and Home Nursing Agency staff have demonstrated the extent to which nursing can influence health care service delivery to rural residents. From community and individual family assessments, to outreach, care coordination, and service delivery, this unique project permits students to participate in a comprehensive, rural, community-based educational experience.

Table 5–1
Rural Nursing Center Student Experiences and Outcomes

Strategies/Activities	Student Competencies/Outcome
Health Promotion/Disease Prevention	
Student participation in the following:	
Health fairs: population and/or topic specific (e.g., elderly, children, pregnancy, diabetes, foot care, mobile mammography, or dental care).	Acquire skill and confidence in developing and delivering health promotion programs.
Immunization clinics/flu campaigns.	Gain ease in communicating with rural residents, school officials, teachers, students, and other community stakeholders.
Schools—family health education nights, teen support groups.	
Community/civic organization.	
CPR/first aid classes.	Develop confidence and skill in providing nursing care.
Parenting classes.	Understand and value relationships that develop among rural providers.
Substance abuse prevention programs.	
Agricultural extension/farm safety programs.	
Home Visits and Individual/Group Contacts at Rural Centers	
Wellness/illness care.	Benefit from supervised clinical activity and the mentor relationship.
Intensive/episodic visits.	Gain confidence in making decisions related to health/illness conditions and assessment skills.
Home environment/safety assessments.	
	Increase effectiveness and confidence related to communicating with clients and families.
	Value lifelong learning.
Care Coordination/Multidisciplinary Collaboration	
Client advocacy.	Develop understanding of managed collaboration to facilitate care and cut costs.
Care planning.	
Participation in nursing center work groups (e.g., clinical practice, telecommunications, research, and evaluation).	Gain flexibility in interpersonal skills and multiple nursing roles.
	Increase appreciation of many disciplines.
Use of community resources.	Understand and value the role of family and friends in achieving patient outcomes.
Multiorganization/multidisciplinary collaboration.	Gain experience in communicating with third-party payers/managed care providers.

Table 5–1 (Continued)

Strategies/Activities	Student Competencies/Outcome
Community Assessment and Analysis Framework identification. Analysis of existing data (e.g., U.S. census data, local, regional, state reports, mortality, morbidity, vital and demographic statistics). Household, door-to-door surveys. Key informant interviews, focused conversations with community representatives (e.g., clergy, local merchants, realtors, borough/village officials). Focus groups/town meetings, using a specific format to elicit perceptions of community health needs.	Gain knowledge of secondary sources. Develop community research skills. Combine/synthesize data analysis to determine community health needs and resources. Identify and understand rural interrelationships and networks. Gain knowledge of values and mores of rural culture. Experience development of multidisciplinary action plans. Acculturate to rural community—respect insider/outsider phenomenon. Identify family structure relationships, strengths and needs. Increase poise in leading community groups. Understand and value rural leadership.
Epidemiology/Case Finding Identification of at-risk individual and aggregate client populations. Work with primary, secondary, and tertiary models of prevention in the community. Screening and detection programs for chronic conditions.	Understand need and process for documentation and data collection. Increase interpersonal skills to work with center staff as well as clients and families. Gain confidence in decision making related to data collection and utilization of tools. Acquire ease in interacting with community leaders.
Outcomes Evaluation Clinical documentation. Data analysis. Assessment of community response to nursing interventions. Increased familiarity with nursing/management information systems. Participation in quality monitoring. Work with outcome, process, and structure criteria/indicators to evaluate quality of nursing care.	Increase ability to articulate program goals. Gain experience working with clients, physicians, and other health providers to articulate outcomes. Develop ability and appreciation for data analysis and interpretation of outcomes. Understand informatics and technology utilization.

Note: Grateful acknowledgment is extended to the Penn State students enrolled in the Rural Health Nursing course during Fall Semester 1996 for their thoughtful comments and contributions in the development of this table.

The integration that must occur and the collaborative relationships that must be developed if health outcomes are to be achieved beckon students and faculty to participate at levels that they may not otherwise encounter. Table 5–1 outlines the scope of activities, competencies, and outcomes associated with placement in a rural nursing center.

SUMMARY

In this chapter, several exciting opportunities and challenges for student practice in a rural nursing center have been presented. Nurses are particularly well positioned to be integrally involved in the delivery of rural health care services and in the shaping of rural health policies. The placement of nursing students in rural settings offers a unique opportunity to kindle in students the interest and enthusiasm for rural nursing practice. Attracting and retaining nurses to work in rural areas where there are significant shortages of available nursing personnel can be greatly facilitated by student clinical experiences in rural settings. Nursing students at all levels of educational preparation (associate degree through nurse practitioner) can benefit from emphasis on rural health content in their nursing school curricula.

REFERENCES

Bandman, E., & Bandman, B. (1995). *Critical thinking in nursing* (2nd ed.). Norwalk, CT: Appleton & Lange.

Barger, S. E. (1991). The nursing center: A model for rural nursing practice. *Nursing & Health Care, 12*(6), 290–294.

Barnett, J. S., & Bigbee, J. L. (1991). Nursing centers: One approach to rural health. In A. Bushy (Ed.), *Rural nursing* (Vol. 2, pp. 166–178). Newbury Park, CA: Sage.

Bigbee, J. L. (1993). The uniqueness of rural nursing. In J. Anderson (Ed.), *The Nursing Clinics of North America, 28*(1), pp. 131–144.

Buerhaus, P. I. (1996). Opportunities, anxieties, and challenges for nursing. *Nursing Policy Forum, 2*(4), 7.

Bushy, A. (1992). Rural determinants in family health: Considerations for community nursing. In A. Bushy (Ed.), *Rural nursing* (Vol. 1, pp. 133–145). Newbury Park, CA: Sage.

Corrigan, C. (1992). Implementing rural preceptorships in baccalaureate nursing education. In P. Winstead-Fry, J. C. Tiffany, R. V. Shippie-Rice (Eds.), *Rural health nursing*, (pp. 333–358). New York: National League for Nursing Press.

Kagawa-Singer, M., Pelusi, J. L., & Underwood, S. M. (1995). *On the frontier: The challenge and rewards of rural nursing research.* Triangle Park, NC: Glaxo.

Lee, H. J. (1993). Rural elderly individuals: Strategies for delivery of nursing care. In J. Anderson (Ed.), *The Nursing Clinics of North America, 28*(1), 219–230.

Lenz, C. L., & Edwards, J. (1992). Nurse-managed primary care: Tapping the rural community power base. *Journal of Nursing Administration, 22*(9), 57–61.

Marczynski-Music, K. N. (1994). *Health care solutions: Designing community-based systems that work.* San Francisco: Jossey-Bass.

Pennsylvania Office of Rural Health News (1994). University Park, PA.

Porter-O'Grady, T. (1994). Building partnerships in health care: Creating whole systems changes. *Nursing & Health Care, 15*(1), 34–38.

Richmond, F. K., & Steketee, M. W. (1995). *Pennsylvania partnerships for children: The state of the child in Pennsylvania.* Harrisburg, PA.

Stratton, T. D., Dunkin, J. W., & Juhl, N. (1993). How states respond to the rural nursing shortage, *Nursing & Health Care, 14*(5), 238–243.

Tymann, B., & Orloff, T. M. (1995). *Rural health: An evolving system of accessible services.* Washington, DC: National Governors' Association.

U.S. Bureau of the Census. (1990). *Statistical Abstract of the United States.* Washington, DC: U.S. Bureau of the Census.

Yawn, B. P. (1994). Rural medical practice: Present and future. In B. P. Yawn, A. Bushy, & R. A. Yawn (Eds.), *Rural medicine: Current issues and concepts* (pp. 1–16). Thousand Oaks, CA: Sage.

6

Research and Collaboration

The Key to New Graduates in Home Care

Barbara White
Karin Conway
Kelly Gallant

Collaboration between the academic and practice setting was key to the vision of hiring new graduates in Home HealthONE (recently renamed Columbia Home Care), a large Denver-based home care agency. A conscious effort was made to lay collaborative groundwork between a private university and a large integrated health care system in Denver, Colorado. The academic-practice partnership developed over three years. The emerging partnership moved from an informal collaboration to a recognized Academic-Practice Council (APC). Through the APC, nurse leader colleagues from the university and the health care system continue to gather monthly to promote collaboration between academic education and professional practice by enhancing the education of nursing students, improving outcomes in the practice settings, and being proactive in health care reform.

The authors wish to gratefully acknowledge the following colleagues for their many contributions to the success of the New Graduate Home Care Program: Nicole Bobo, RN, MSN, Assistant Professor, Department of Nursing, Regis University; Sara Jarrett, RN, MA, MS, Assistant Professor, Department of Nursing, Regis University; Lou Anne Epperson, RN, MSN, Clinical Director, NurseFinders; former Director of Patient Care Services, Home HealthONE.

SHARED ISSUES

In early 1995, Home HealthONE was experiencing unique staffing challenges. Over the preceding year, the number of staff RNs increased by 42 percent, and more nurses were needed to meet the exploding growth in number of visits. Initially Home HealthONE had no difficulty hiring staff from a pool of nurses with at least one year of home care experience. However, as the hiring needs increased, the availability of experienced home care nurses diminished, and managers were compelled to hire nurses without such experience. Home HealthONE, like other home care agencies in the city, never hired new graduates. Home care required a minimum of one year of acute care experience, preferably medical/surgical. Nurse leaders came to APC seeking innovative ways to increase RN staffing.

Nursing faculty at Regis University were concerned about the changing practice settings for new graduates. At the same time, goal-oriented senior students asked how they could begin their practice in home care rather than in the traditional acute care hospital setting. With available positions, it was usual for a hospital nurse manager to hire graduate nurses who had spent their senior advanced practicum in the manager's unit. Home care managers, however, were firm in their belief that new hires must have "experience" before engaging in the autonomous practice of the home care setting. Faculty came to the APC seeking innovative ways to prepare new graduates for community based and home care practice immediately on graduation.

The reality of the changing health care environment impacted the issue of new graduates in home care. There were no positions open for new graduates within the hospital. The home care agency was desperate for new staff. It became evident that a shared dilemma existed. APC determined the best way to match patient needs with available quality RNs was to initiate a competency-based new graduate program. To provide a sound educational base for practice, the university agreed to develop and offer elective courses in home care nursing to senior nursing students. The home care agency agreed to develop and implement a pilot New Graduate Home Care Program (NGHCP) with a commitment to hire two new graduates. APC formed a task force to develop, implement, and evaluate the program.

HOME CARE COMPETENCY ASSESSMENT

The scope of nursing practice in home care is broader and more autonomous than in the acute care setting. Lack of access to immediate human and technological support systems, chaotic home environments, complex decision making, coordination of care, and a wide repertoire of assessment and therapeutic interventions present the home care nurse with multiple stressors. To develop the program, the first essential initial step was to survey expert home care nurses and to delineate knowledge, skills, and competencies needed in home care practice. The results would be the foundation of curriculum development for novice home care nurses.

A survey tool was developed based on 27 topics or skill sets necessary for proficient home care nursing practice (Table 6–1). Topics were determined by asking home care nursing staff what skills were necessary to perform their job, by reviewing home care nurse job descriptions, and by asking home care nurse managers what skills they perceive reflected proficient home care practice. An example of some of the topics is given in Figure 6–1. The survey was distributed to expert home care RNs (greater than one year home care experience), novice home care RNs (less than one year home care experience), and hospital RNs with no home care experience. Nurses were asked to assess each skill set based on their knowledge, skill, and comfort in practice.

Utilizing a convenience sample of over 150 nurses, responses were analyzed according to the respondent's age, educational background, nursing experience, and home care expertise. Data analysis for overall perception of the 27 topics by educational preparation is summarized in Figure 6–2. Courses were developed and offered at both the undergraduate and graduate level based on previous educational preparation of nurses. Analysis of data according to years of experience in health care is also indicated in Figure 6–2. Results indicated that RNs with minimal to no home care experience perceived their overall knowledge as high, whereas RNs with one year or more of home care experience perceived their knowledge as lower than those with minimal or no experience. Analysis of topics led to the development of curriculum content for the NGHCP. Topics rated low in "knowledge" were included in the theory portion of the home care nursing courses. Topics that represented a low percentage of responses in the "skillful" or "comfortable" areas were emphasized in the practicum portion of the home care nursing courses.

Table 6–1
Skill Sets

1. Assessing resources.
2. Communication with physicians.
3. Interdisciplinary teamwork.
4. Working with third-party payer requirements.
5. Planning frequency and duration of home visits.
6. Education techniques.
7. Contracting for mutual goals.
8. Patient's responsibility in self-care.
9. Assessing family.
10. Assessing the community.
11. Assessing home.
12. Problem solving/critical thinking.
13. Utilizing management.
14. Physical assessment.
15. IV venipuncture skills.
16. Documentation requirements.
17. Ethical considerations.
18. Legal issues.
19. Lab values.
20. Pharmacology.
21. Drug/food interactions.
22. Technical equipment skills.
23. Assessing age-specific needs.
24. Wound care.
25. Communication skills.
26. Alternative treatment.
27. Psychosocial needs.

HOME CARE NURSING COURSES

Regis faculty utilized the survey data to develop elective courses in home care nursing. Students interested in immediate home care practice after graduation were informed of the pilot program and advised to take the home care electives offered in the spring of 1995. The theory-based course entitled *Topics in Clinical Nursing: Theoretical Concepts in Home Care* (3 semester hours) provided an overview of contemporary home

Figure 6–1
Homecare Competency Survey

Skill Set	Examples	Knowledgeable*	Skillful†	Comfortable‡
1. Assessing community resources.	Meals on Wheels. Transportation. Hospice.	————	————	————
4. Working with third party payer.	Accessing case management nurse. HMO's philosophy.	————	————	————
5. Planning frequency and duration of home visits according to treatment plan.	Time management. Setting goals and setting time frames.	————	————	————
11. Assessing environment and home safety.	Is patient safe to remain in home by self?	————	————	————

* I understand the theory and/or rationale for this topic's importance in home health care.
† I have the ability to perform or carry out the topic independently in the home care setting.
‡ I feel confident in being able to perform or carry out the topic independently and safely in the home care setting.

Figure 6–2
Home Care Comparison
(Overall Average Perception)

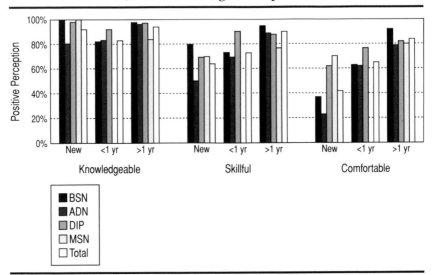

Figure 6–3
Home Care Nursing Courses

Topics in Clinical Nursing: Theoretical Concepts in Home Care

Course Description: This 3 SH theory course introduces the senior student to home care as a nursing speciality. Students explore the roles and function of the home care nurse, identify patient populations served by home care, and discuss pertinent patient care management issues. Home care concepts including theoretical frameworks, standards of practice, interdisciplinary teams, ethical and legal issues, reimbursement, and home care delivery systems are analyzed. Selected home care client exemplars, home visit parameters, and clinical competencies are discussed. Students participate in an observational experience in the home care setting.

Objectives

1. Describe the roles and functions of the home care nurse.
2. Explain how the structure of home care delivery systems influence nursing practice.
3. Compare conceptual frameworks used in home care nursing.
4. Articulate how age, disease process, culture, family structure, and health beliefs influence health and illness behaviors of patients in the home setting.
5. Identify major health concerns/risks for targeted home care populations.
6. Examine concepts and issues relevant to home care nursing.
7. Identify clinical competencies required of the novice home care nurse.
8. Relate nursing research to practice in the home care environment.

Topics in Clinical Nursing: Home Care Practicum

Course Description: This 2 SH clinical practicum is designed to provide the senior student with 90 hours of preceptored clinical experience in a home care agency. Practicum will focus on clinical competencies required of the novice home care nurse. Seminars provide an opportunity to dialogue with other students, share clinical issues, and integrate theoretical knowledge. Reflective journaling and completion of clinical objectives are required.

Clinical Objectives

1. Perform in the role of novice home care nurse as defined by selected clinical competencies.
2. Incorporate professional and ethical behavior in clinical practice.
3. Integrate nursing theory and research into clinical practice.
4. Apply the nursing process to the care of home care patients.
5. Utilize community resources in meeting the needs of patients and families.
6. Integrate knowledge of aging, disease process, culture, and health beliefs in the planning of nursing care.
7. Collaborate with and coordinate care by other health care providers.
8. Assess own learning needs and utilize appropriate resources to promote professional growth.

care issues and topics. The clinical course entitled *Topics in Clinical Nursing: Home Care Practicum* was developed as a clinical course that required students to complete 90 contact hours in a home care agency under the direct supervision of an approved preceptor. Faculty facilitated the learning process by integrating concepts during 16 additional hours of clinical seminar and by frequent interaction with the students and preceptors. Students were responsible for meeting home care clinical objectives as well as personally defined learning goals. Course descriptions and objectives are presented in Figure 6–3.

NEW GRADUATE HOME CARE PROGRAM

Program development and planning for new graduates to enter home care upon graduation occurred over nine months. Administrative dialogue and support were a crucial part of the program approval process. Several meetings were held to discuss issues and implications from all perspectives. A formal proposal, including program overview, objectives, and a proposed weekly clinical and didactic schedule, was drafted and presented to nursing administration and human resources in the health care system. The Colorado State Board of Nursing was contacted to discuss rules and regulations regarding the new program. As the program began to take shape, documents were circulated to the Regis nursing program director, the Home HealthONE nursing administrator, and other key stakeholders for feedback and approval. Collaborative processes, which had been a part of the program since its inception, continued throughout.

The 12-month NGHCP, divided into two 6-month phases, was designed to familiarize the new graduate with home care concepts and to assist the new graduate with clearly delineated clinical experiences to promote competency and professional growth. The goal for the new graduate was to become a novice home care nurse. During the first phase, the graduate functioned under the direct supervision of a carefully selected preceptor with daily feedback and weekly competency goals. During the first few weeks of the program, the learner and preceptor shared a patient case load and met weekly to discuss client needs, set priorities, coordinate with other team members, and reflect on critical learning. Clinical benchmarks for Phase I are summarized in Figure 6–4. During the second phase, the new graduate functioned

Figure 6–4
New Graduate Home Care Program Phase I (Weeks 1–26) Clinical Benchmarks

The goal of Phase I is to assist the new graduate in becoming knowledgeable and competent in the role of an RN novice home care case manager.

Week 1	Completes new hire orientation. Meets preceptor, team leader, and supervisor. Observes admissions, Home Health Aide (HHA), and RN scheduling. Observes preceptor in field focusing on organizational skills.
Weeks 2–3	"Buddies" with preceptor. Emphasis on physical assessment, venipuncture, wound care, catheterization, and documentation. Learns daily functions and communication channels. Obtains daily feedback from preceptor. Meets weekly with preceptor and team leader to review goals.
Weeks 4–9	Shares a patient case load and continues to meet weekly with preceptor to discuss clinical needs of patients, priority setting, and appropriate communication with the team. Emphasis on blood sugar finger sticks; staple and suture removal; open and discharge documentation; recertification; HHA care and supervision; diabetic, respiratory, and cardiac case management.
Weeks 10–15	Manages case load of 5 patients. Emphasis on total health assessment; resources and referral; physician communication; and care plan management. Continues to meet weekly for one hour with preceptor and team leader.
Weeks 16–21	Manages simple IV cases in addition to small case load. Emphasis on venipuncture; PICC, subclavian, and central venous catheter lines; blood draws from lines; access ports and needleless systems; multilumen catheter care. Continues to meet weekly for one-half hour with preceptor and team leader.
Weeks 22–26	Carries a full patient case load. Completes check-off of competencies. Emphasis on team building; ethical and legal issues; alternative treatment modalities; performance standards; competent home care nursing practice. Meets with preceptor and team leader every two weeks.

under the supervision of a home care team leader with consultation from the nursing supervisor. During Phase II, the new graduate functioned in the home care role carrying a full case load of patients.

The cost analysis, which was critical to final approval of the NGHCP, focused on Phase I, the most expensive phase of the program. It was anticipated that during the second phase, the new graduate would be more productive in terms of the number of visits, and program cost would greatly decrease. Phase I projected costs per new graduate were based on nonproductive time for the new graduate, preceptor, and team leader. Nonproductive time was defined as time spent in nonpatient contact activities. New graduates received the same initial three-week intensive preceptored experience as any home care new hire; therefore, initial orientation cost was the same. During the next six weeks, both new graduate and preceptor were considered to have 0.5 nonproductive time. Over the remaining weeks of Phase I, the new graduate and preceptor spent less time in conference activities. Projected total nonproductive hours for Phase I was 368:175 for the new graduate, 175 for the preceptor, and 18 for the team leader. Projected cost per graduate was $6,672. The new graduate salary rate was $2.75 less than other home care new hires who have one to two years of acute care clinical experience. This salary difference provided a cost savings of $5,720 per graduate. Therefore, total Phase I cost was projected at less than $1,000.

Hiring criteria were developed jointly by the home care agency and the university. Only BSN Regis applicants were considered for the pilot program. Applicants were required to have successfully completed the home care elective courses and had to present two letters of recommendation, one from a medical-surgical faculty member and one from a community health faculty member. Faculty was asked to address the graduate's critical thinking, communication, assessment, and therapeutic intervention competencies. Applicants submitted a portfolio to Home HealthONE that included a summary of their scholarly work, transcript with GPA, and an essay describing their home care goals and reflections. Applicants were interviewed, as are all potential new hires. Two new graduates applied and were hired in October 1995. Selection criteria were based on motivation, competency, and evidence of leadership ability. Candidates were drawn to home care based on the autonomy of this nursing practice. They recognized that in some cases, the home care nurse may be the only contact with the patient and the primary link to the physician and other health team members. The new graduates had confidence in their assessment skills, recognizing that they would have to determine the appropriate level of care for clients. They felt comfortable with time management, organizational skills, and critical thinking. In addition, they were comfortable delegating nonnurse tasks to other team members. Both demonstrated effective communication, a vital characteristic for the eventual coordination of the entire multidisciplinary team. They also demonstrated the ability to provide clear and concise directions to clients and were effective teachers.

Preceptors, who were chosen from the staff, demonstrated proficiency in all aspects of client care. The preceptors were recognized leaders among their peers, had previous preceptor experience, and received excellent annual performance appraisals. Regis faculty and agency nursing directors met with the preceptors prior to commencing the program to orient them, explain the competencies, and delineate the unique responsibilities of this new mentoring role. Since Phase I was a 6-month commitment, preceptors had to be participants who felt comfortable with the support structures and parameters.

Preceptors soon became the new graduates' strong and supportive mentors. During the first few weeks, they served as advocates for the new graduates as the program was presented and discussed at nursing staff team meetings. Preceptors taught new skills, reinforced the principles and rationale of practice, engaged the new graduates in scientific inquiry, and gradually encouraged independent decision making. Preceptors were responsible for assuring the new graduates a broad-based, diverse case load. They evaluated and signed off on competencies and gave continual feedback on case and practice issues. Examples of goals, interventions, and competencies for Week 1 are given in Figure 6–5, and for Weeks 4 through 9 in Figure 6–6.

During the first phase of the program, several support structures were implemented to monitor progress and deal with issues as they appeared. The committed Regis faculty who had developed and taught the home care courses, remained available to meet and dialogue with the participants. This faculty provided a listening ear when the new graduates were overwhelmed or frustrated. Issues were always directed back to the new graduate, preceptor, and team leader to manage, but this outside voice provided balance and wisdom. Another faculty provided preceptors with guidance and support as needed. At times, phone conversations were sufficient to assure comfort and progress. At other times, lunch meetings were arranged to deal with clinical mentoring issues. This faculty also interacted with the nursing supervisor, team leaders, and the entire nursing staff team to clarify program objectives, amplify competencies, and support both preceptor and new graduate roles. The APC home care task force continued to meet quarterly to discuss program issues and to monitor progress in clinical benchmarks.

New graduates progressed more quickly than anticipated. By Week 16, four months into the program, both new graduates had completed all competencies and had exceeded the six-month benchmarks. They were carrying full case loads and rarely needed preceptor advice. Over the four months, they had been transformed from new graduates to novice home care nurses to competent practitioners. Through consensus of the preceptors, team leaders, and nursing supervisor, the new graduates moved into Phase II of the program two months early and began interacting

Figure 6–5
Orientation Goals for Week One

Goals	Interventions
1. Become familiar with HealthONE's programs and services to include benefits and other health and safety topics.	1. Attend HealthONE orientation and review employee handbook.
2. Learn the role of the Admission RN and how information shared between Adm. RN and caregiver is important in delivering patient care.	2. Observe and interact with Adm. RN.
3. Identify scheduling patterns and importance of weekly schedule.	3. Observe and interact with RN schedule.
4. Identify how to call and what information HHA schedulers need in order to staff HHA services.	4. Observe and interact with HHA schedule.
5. Learn how to complete lab slips.	5. Complete lab slip for preceptor.
6. Learn where to find forms, supplies, mailbox, paperwork turn-in box, and revisit turn-in box.	6. Take tour and observe preceptor in finding these items.
7. Learn how to activate and use voice mail.	7. With the help of preceptor, set up VM prompts and listen to messages.
8. Identify proper bag technique.	8. Observe bag technique demonstration and use bag technique in the field.
9. Learn to complete time card.	9. Observe and participate in class presentation and complete own time card with assistance from preceptor.

Figure 6–5 (*Continued*)

Competencies	Follow-Up Needed
Completion of Lab Order Forms	
Bag Technique	

Bag Technique—Performance Skill Checklist

Criterion Behavior	Acceptable	Comments
Sets bag on hard surface on a paper towel.	_____	_____
Accesses own soap and towel from outside pocket of bag.	_____	_____
Washes hands before opening the bag.	_____	_____
Lays supplies needed for visit out of bag all at once on a paper towel.	_____	_____
Cleans thermometer and stethoscope with alcohol before using.	_____	_____
Uses probe cover on thermometer.	_____	_____
Returns supplies back to bag when finished with them.	_____	_____
Washes hands before leaving the home.	_____	_____
States when bags must be cleaned and where to document this.	_____	_____
Bag is stored in a clean box in the car or trunk.	_____	_____
Properly stores discipline-specific items in bag.	_____	_____

Figure 6–6
Orientation Goals for Weeks Four through Nine

Goals	Interventions
1. Shares a case load with preceptor and maintains preceptor's productivity.	1. Completes 10–13 patient visits independently.
2. By Week 9, completes an "open" independently.	2. "Opens" a medical management patient independently.
3. Demonstrates knowledge on how to complete a recertification.	3. With minimal supervision, completes a recert.
4. By the end of Week 9, independently completes a HHA supervisory visit.	4. Completes a minimum of three supervisory visits of a HHA with preceptor prior to completing one independently.
5. Demonstrates knowledge of how to complete a discharge.	5. Completes discharge paperwork.

(Continued)

Figure 6–6 (*Continued*)

Goals	Interventions
6. Demonstrates knowledge of DM management of a patient.	6. Carries a DM patient demonstrating appropriate management and attends Center of Diabetes Management for observation.
7. Demonstrates knowledge of Resp/Cardiac management of a patient.	7. Carries a Resp/Cardiac patient demonstrating appropriate management and attends Resp/Cardiac clinic.
8. Demonstrates the ability to manage a small caseload independently.	8. Prioritizes and communicates patient needs. Able to work with interdisciplinary team members.
9. Understands roles of other caregivers/disciplines in the home.	9. Spends time in field with each discipline and verbalizes roles of each to preceptor.

Competencies	Follow-Up Needed
Finger Stick Blood Sugar	
Staple Removal	
Suture Removal	
Open Paperwork	
HHA Plan of Care	
HHA Supervisory Visit	
Recertification	
Discharge	

Suture Removal—Performance Skill Checklist

Criterion Behavior	Acceptable	Comments
Washes hands.	_____	_____
Prepares required equipment.	_____	_____
Identifies patient.	_____	_____
Assesses wound for readiness for removal of sutures.	_____	_____
Positions and prepares patient.		
A. Sitting or reclined position depending on sutured area.	_____	_____
B. Explain procedure.	_____	_____
Removes sutures using sterile scissors and tweezers.	_____	_____
Examines wound for drainage, warmth, swelling, dehiscence, etc.	_____	_____
Applies steri strips, if necessary.	_____	_____
Disposes of sutures properly.	_____	_____
Documents.	_____	_____

with team leaders, rather than preceptors, on a consistent basis. The six-month evaluation, completed by the nursing supervisor and used as a standard for all new hire nurses, documented above-average performance in all areas of practice.

PROGRAM SUCCESS

Several factors account for the overwhelming success of this New Graduate Home Care Program. Through program evaluation, new graduate interviews, preceptor discussions, and task force dialogue, the success of the program was evident. Program success was particularly due to new graduate commitment and motivation. These specific graduates knew without a doubt that their career goal was home care practice. They were confident in their beginning skill levels and they believed in their ability to become competent home care practitioners. Their BSN education had prepared them to think critically, communicate effectively, and intervene therapeutically. They admitted that, even at times when they questioned their capabilities in response to other nurses' doubts and fears, they knew they could "learn it and do it." Preceptors' mentoring skills and dedication to program success were crucial. Although hesitant and resistant at first, the preceptors willingly undertook the time commitment necessary to overcome their concerns about the quality of care provided by new graduates without experience. Once engaged, they became champions for these new graduates in this new role. They were strong and powerful advocates to other staff who gradually became open and willing to support the innovative program. Rigorous education for the new graduates and in-depth understanding of clinical mentoring for the preceptors were critical for program success. The theory and clinical practicum experience were vital to prepare new graduates for this unique practice specialty. Clear delineation of weekly goals, competencies, and benchmarks were necessary for the new graduate to focus on clinical growth and professional development. The nursing supervisor, who admits to being very skeptical at first, spent many extra hours writing competencies and administratively overseeing the program. Administrative support, both financial and time resources, were imperative for the program approval and successful outcomes. And finally, without the trust and collaboration through the APC, the program never would have become a reality.

Collaboration between educators and practitioners can result in powerful outcomes. Nursing roles no longer follow the descriptors of the recent past. New graduates entering the practice setting do not find "typical" new graduate positions. Nursing faculties are creatively defining content as curricula are redesigned to focus on community-based practice. Collaboration can significantly impact on both academic nursing education and clinical practice.

SECTION III

Complementary Paths

Building Collaborative Relationships in a
Community-Based Health Care System

7

Associate Degree and Baccalaureate Degree Nursing Education

Finding Complementary Paths in a Population-Focused Health Care System

Andrea Mengel
Gloria Donnelly

The universe is change; our life is what our thoughts make it.
Marcus Aurelius Antonius

These words, written almost two thousand years ago by a Roman philosopher, mirror the state of the contemporary health care system, nursing practice, and nursing education. We are in the midst of an unprecedented change in health care driven by the demographic engine, the failure of a tertiary care based system to deliver cost-effective care, the rise of managed health care controlled largely by insurers and corporations who purchase health care, and the challenge of providing care to the more than 40 million uninsured and underserved in this nation. Knowing that the changes occurring in health care are a national phenomenon is comforting since all the constituencies of health care and health professions education are facing the same issues. At the same time, the constant and pressing changes mean that each of us must accept the responsibility for creating harmony in a reordered health care system. Nurses especially need to think themselves into harmonious relationships with each other and with other health care disciplines. This chapter will explore the impact of changes in health care on the practice and education of nurses at the associate degree and baccalaureate levels in a population-focused health care system.

Table 7–1 summarizes changes in the health care delivery system that dramatically change the context for nursing education and practice. The changes in the health care system alter the context for nursing education and practice. Inherent in these changes is the shift to an emphasis on economics with the prominent values of efficiency, effectiveness, and the documentation of value gained for dollars spent. The accompanying shift to a primary care, health promotion orientation forces us to rethink what associate degree and baccalaureate education have considered their traditional turfs of knowledge and practice. Associate degree nursing programs were originally developed to prepare the first line, bedside nurse for acute care settings. Baccalaureate nursing programs have traditionally included education and practice in community-based or public health nursing practice, with an emphasis on determining the needs of aggregate communities (e.g., schools, neighborhoods, towns, and cities). Now that hospitals are closing and downsizing, what will be the role of the associate degree nursing graduate? Now that the aggregate and primary care is the focus, how will baccalaureate programs change to emphasize these areas? Can the two programs coexist and provide smooth articulation paths that match changing health care needs and the system?

Table 7–1
Trends in Health Care Delivery Systems

From	To
Acute inpatient care	Life-span care
Treating illness	Maintaining health
Focus on the individual	Focus on the aggregates/population
Product of care orientation	Value of care orientation
Number of admissions to hospital	Number of lives covered (capitation)
Managing organizations	Managing networks
Managing departments	Managing markets
Coordinating services	Documenting quality and outcomes

Note: Ideas in this table were summarized from a presentation by William Warfed, PhD, RN, at the meeting of the Council of Baccalaureate and Higher Degree Programs in Portland, Oregon, 1994.

ACUTE CARE, HOME CARE, POPULATION-BASED CARE: THE DIFFERENCES AND THE NEEDS

As patients are discharged from the hospital at faster rates and with continuing care needs, care that historically occurred in hospitals is now occurring in the home, which for the nurse is an environment of uncertainty. Examples of acute care delivered in the home are wound assessment, dressing changes, pain management, and life support care for patients with chronic illnesses, such as AIDS, COPD, and kidney disease. Acquiring the knowledge and skill base to deliver care in the home is a basic expectation for all nursing students; arguably, home care is an extension of the bedside expertise required of all nursing students. Thus home care is well within the purview of the associate degree nursing graduate although it differs in the acuity level and complexity of patient care that needs to be delivered in the absence of the hospital's structured environment rich in backup and supports for the caregiver. Further, since much of continuing care is thrust onto families, nurses must function as experts in assessing, managing, and teaching families. These patients and families need caregivers not only with the technical skill base but with a breadth of knowledge about how families from diverse cultural groups function in health and illness.

In addition to continuing care in the home, there is a shift in focus on the needs of the aggregate or the defined population. Assessing aggregates for health risks and planning care accordingly is the essence of population-focused care. For example, in the northwestern section of Philadelphia, there are many old homes containing lead-based paint and plaster. Children living in this area are at high risk for lead poisoning. Nurses in a nurse managed health center in the area worked with the Department of Health to establish a lead poisoning screening site. They also worked with the Environmental Protection Agency to provide low-technology lead abatement (cleanup) in the homes to prevent further problems.

In addition to focusing care on obvious needs (as in the case of lead poisoning), nurses must work with the defined population in identifying needs. For example, residents of an urban minority housing project with a high crime rate met with public health nurses to plan for their health care needs. Their highest priority was not childhood immunizations, prenatal care, or hypertension screening. Instead, they wanted cardiopulmonary resuscitation training for residents who were overwhelmed by the violence and drug overdoses affecting their children. They believed that paramedic response time was slow to "the projects." This was a test for the caregivers, who needed to place the priorities of the community first instead of imposing their own health care agenda.

Whether nursing practice is focused on the individual in the home or on the aggregate with a health risk, the ecology of the service area needs to be a prime factor in the delivery of care. What works in an older city of ethnic neighborhoods, such as Chicago or Philadelphia, may not work in a newer city like Phoenix or Dallas. Baccalaureate nursing programs have used in-depth community assessment to determine the character of the community and the shape that care delivery should take. Associate degree educators, cognizant that many of their graduates will deliver care in the home, are designing educational experiences to heighten the awareness of the nature of the community and its resources. For example, associate degree nursing students in the Zip Code 19130 Project learn to develop partnerships with community-based agencies. The project focuses on extending existing services rather than on creating new services. As described in Chapter 17, the students discovered that many residents are unaware of their neighborhood's resources or are unable to access them without assistance. The students are developing ways to connect people with existing services. In the process, students are learning collaboration skills and extending care to those in need.

In Philadelphia, associate degree and baccalaureate nursing educators are finding complementary paths as they reinvent nursing education at both levels to meet the needs of the changing health care delivery system. This complementarity is fueled by the collegial relationships and mutual respect of nursing leaders in both associate degree and baccalaureate nursing programs. This unique collaboration is further supported because both levels of nursing education have an opportunity to redesign nursing care that will be increasingly delivered outside the hospital and in homes, schools, churches, and other nontraditional settings. Urban and rural poor Americans, historically underserved, have been the primary beneficiaries of public health initiatives and public health nursing. Their lack of access to health care continues to be a considerable problem that might be addressed by all levels of nursing education. The current and continuing emphasis on cost-effective care, the nursing care needs of home care clients, aggregates with specific health risks, and the underserved present challenges as urgent as addressing the primary care needs of the general population. Who can deliver the highest quality, most cost-effective care? Traditionally, there has been little difference in the starting salaries of associate degree and baccalaureate educated nurses. Further, hospital staff nurses have traditionally earned more than public health nurses. Given the lack of differentiation in salaries, nurse educators should focus on designing levels and foci of care for graduates of each program type that most effectively serve the population's need for seamless, humanistic care. We need to focus less on the traditional meaning of the degree and more on the purpose of the basic preparation at each level. It is also essential to decide what can be delegated to unlicensed personnel.

WHAT ARE THE IMPLICATIONS FOR NURSING?

As health care changes, the nursing curriculum will change. The changing health care system needs workers who are educated, flexible, and committed to lifelong learning. What level of preparation and how many nurses are needed remain up for discussion; however, there is no dispute that community-based care is the future and that it requires different skills than hospital-based care. Educators agree that too few minorities are entering nursing and too few of those who do seek advanced degrees.

Historically, both associate degree and baccalaureate nursing education have sought a balance between liberal and technical education. Both have seen social relevance as part of their mission. Outstanding examples include the public health efforts of baccalaureate educators with immigrant populations and the education of immigrant populations in community colleges. While social relevance remains a deeply held value in both programs, questions arise about the appropriate balance between technology and liberal studies and the traditional structure of upper and lower division nursing building on a liberal base. Much more work needs to be done on the outcomes associated with building on liberal education as well as on the restructuring of both programs. Education in colleges and universities is compartmentalized by discipline while nursing practice requires integrated knowledge. A practicing nurse must consider the client's physiological and psychosocial needs, the legal and ethical parameters for practice, resources available, and other complex factors not learned in a single course. How does this information get integrated now and are there better ways to synthesize information to improve practice? With the accessibility of information and the knowledge explosion, we must rethink our approach to education. Curricula must adapt to rapid change and be flexible. Knowledge has exploded so significantly in the past 10 years that a mapped curriculum, with objectives cross-referenced for every course, no longer works. The curricula needs to focus on teaching students basic principles about care and teaching them to access information in a variety of ways, traditional or technical, so that students can access the information they need to solve problems. Those who learn to learn will make their mark.

HOW CAN WE PLAN FOR THE FUTURE?

This we know: Changes in the health care system are challenging the way we think about nursing education and nursing practice. Negotiating our way through these changes and strengthening nursing's position in the reordered health care system will test our cohesion and flexibility. We will be successful if we build on our strengths and maximize our resources.

One strength is the articulated career ladder. Community colleges have traditionally been attractive to minority populations. In Pennsylvania, the majority of minority students who access higher education do so through the community college system. The low cost, along with the availability of remedial courses for students whose secondary schools did not adequately prepare them for college, is likely to ensure continuation of this market. Approximately 25 percent of Americans represent ethnic minority populations, yet only 10 percent of registered nurses represent ethnic minority populations. More troubling is the number of registered nurses from ethnic minorities with advanced degrees. While 7 percent of white nurses hold a graduate degree in nursing, less than 1 percent of the nurses in any ethnic minority group hold a graduate nursing degree. Education of a diverse workforce hinges on community colleges, which will continue to be the entry point for many ethnic minorities. In addition, as college costs rise and more need is financed by educational loans, an increasing number of middle-class families are expected to choose community colleges. Community colleges have provided social mobility for these students and articulation models have enhanced professional mobility. This social and professional mobility is part of the American dream, and nursing is to be commended for providing opportunities for advancement. With an ethnically diverse workforce, nursing will be better able to provide culturally sensitive health care. This should enhance our ability to collaborate with individuals and communities when delivering population-based care.

We believe that there are complementary roles for associate degree and baccalaureate and higher degree nurses. Past models of differences may not apply in the changed health care system. The move to community-based care has taught us that nursing curricula derives from practice. Nurses practicing in a community-based health care system will need a different body of knowledge and additional clinical skills.

We are proposing an updated model for nursing education that would build on the strengths of the present model and be efficient, effective, diverse, and agile. It would have multiple exit points (associate degree, baccalaureate, master's, and doctorate), meet population-based local health needs in a circumscribed context, and use assistive personnel to provide lower skilled care. Not all schools of nursing will survive. With the downsizing of acute care and cuts in Medicare and Medicaid, the demand for registered nurses will probably decrease. Only the best, most competitive, agile schools will survive.

As educators, we share the mission of designing learning activities to prepare excellent nurses for the job market. Articulation models for nursing education can assist us to build on our strengths, grafting each level of education on the previous level, creating a more efficient and effective model. Grafting is an apt metaphor for another reason. It symbolizes a commitment to live in harmony and share the same space and resources. Host and graft become a thriving integrated whole. Much remains to be done, but we believe this to be desirable for nursing. Certainly it is achievable, because our life will be what our thoughts make it.

8

Associate and Baccalaureate Degree Preparation for Home Health Care in an Era of Managed Care

Mary Beth Hanner

As the turn of the century draws near, it is interesting to reflect on an article I wrote 10 years ago on undergraduate educational preparation for home health care nursing (Hanner, 1985). After reviewing that article as well as contemplating the events of the past decade and attempting to forecast the future, it is easy to see that many current expected competencies remain essential for entry level nursing practice. Additional skills are required, however, to function in an era in which managed care is rapidly changing the delivery of health services. Health insurance payer groups are doing business with large-scale providers who offer a continuum of health care services linked through integrated networks. A capitated approach to managed care requires a strong emphasis on health promotion and maintenance because the provider gets paid a fixed fee for managing the health of groups. The goals are to keep clients out of expensive acute care settings and to eliminate any unnecessary interventions. In this model, the hospital is a cost, rather than a revenue, center. Therefore, hospital beds are being reduced, creating a need for redeployment of the health care workforce.

Critical nursing competencies within a managed care framework include the management of clinical and cost outcomes. Success will be measured by keeping groups of clients healthy enough so that they don't require expensive treatments or services. For example, physical assessment skills to monitor cardiac status and to identify signs of impending decompensation will still be essential in providing home care for a client with congestive heart failure. However, as home care providers join integrated delivery systems, the number and length of home visits will be scrutinized more carefully 'than ever. The emphasis of the nurse/client interaction will be on the development of a self-monitoring teaching plan so that the client and family are taught to monitor the client's health status and report any deviations from expected parameters; the teaching plan would also focus on dietary modification, medications, activity levels, and other lifestyle changes that will maintain the client's health and functional status.

The majority of registered nurses in practice today were educated in associate degree nursing (ADN) programs; this trend will continue for the foreseeable future based on current enrollment patterns in schools of nursing. The emphasis in most ADN programs has been on the care of ill clients in structured settings, most commonly hospitals. As hospital beds rapidly dwindle, many questions are being raised as to the educational preparation and the numbers of nurses who will be needed in a restructured health care system. Is there a role for the associate degree nurse? If so, where will this nurse practice? What competencies are essential for associate and baccalaureate degree nurses? How will we differentiate the practice of these nurses?

This chapter will explore educational preparation for home care nursing, an area of practice that is the fastest growing segment of the health care field and is projected to be the setting in which the majority of care to ill clients will be delivered. I believe that roles will exist for nurses from various educational backgrounds, but these roles must be clearly differentiated and access to baccalaureate and higher degrees must continue to be enhanced. Delineation of specific competencies for each stage of practice and assessment of clinical performance outcomes at the end of each educational program would facilitate articulation between nursing programs.

DIFFERENTIATED NURSING PRACTICE IN THE HOME SETTING

The model that will be used to differentiate nursing practice roles was developed through the Healing Web Project in South Dakota (Chapter 9), a collaborative effort among representatives of associate and baccalaureate degree nursing programs and nursing practice settings from six midwestern and western states. Specific competencies for provision of direct care, communication, and management were developed as well as role descriptions for each clinician. The guiding principles of the project related to mutual respect and valuing of all nursing roles and the belief that differentiation of these roles along a continuum of care will help to match the skills of various nurses to the differing needs of the public they serve. The continuum represents associate, primary, and advanced nursing roles; each role increases in complexity yet all practitioners are valued equally. Each nurse is seen as an expert in the role and collaborative practice utilizing all roles is the "whole" of nursing practice (Larson, 1992).

A joint task force of the American Association of Colleges of Nursing, the American Organization of Nurse Executives, and the National Organization for Associate Degree Nursing recently published *A Model for Differentiated Nursing Practice* (AACN, 1995). Three of the conclusions that they endorsed were:

> *The model of differentiated nursing practice and education being implemented by the Healing Web Project is cost-efficient and promotes high quality nursing care across settings and the life span for all consumers of health care and also job satisfaction for nurses.*

> *To ensure nursing as an integral and permanent component of the future health care system, differentiated nursing practice must be implemented in all health care practice settings and differentiated roles must be taught in ADN and BSN education settings as well.*

> *All three integrated nursing roles are necessary to meet the needs of the future health care system, i.e., to provide high quality, comprehensive cost-effective care to all patients, in all settings. (AACN, 1995 p. 15)*

In collaboration with the Visiting Nurse Association in Sioux Falls, the Healing Web Group has now begun to adapt the model for community health nursing practice as shown in Table 8–1 (Larson, Johnson, Holmes, Leuning, & Schuller, 1995). Three of the differentiated community practice competencies will be analyzed in relation to specific role activities of the primary nurse (BSN) and the associate nurse (ADN).

The differentiated competencies more clearly identify the scope of role responsibilities (Table 8–2). The primary nurse functions as an individual and family case manager from preadmission to postdischarge to

Table 8–1
Healing Web Model: Differentiated
Competencies in the Community

Associate Role	Primary Role
Provision of Care	
Assumes responsibility and accountability for direct nursing care and documentation.	Assumes responsibility and accountability for direct care, caregiver effectiveness, and client outcomes.
Communication	
Modifies, implements, and evaluates a teaching plan to restore, maintain, or promote health.	Designs, implements, and evaluates a holistic teaching plan that will maximize the client's potential for quality of life.
Management Skills	
Evaluates client responses and modifies nursing interventions as necessary to meet client needs.	Evaluates progress toward established goals and promotes goal-directed change to meet client needs.

Table 8–2
Role Responsibilities of the Primary and Associate Nurse

Associate Role	Primary Role
Direct care focus.	Individual/family case manager.
Implementation, modification of plan.	Family/home assessment.
Use of critical pathways, care maps, standards of care.	Formulate nursing diagnoses.
	Contracting with family.
Assess common changes in client status: Physiological. Psychological. Social. Environmental.	Develop plans for provision of care, self-monitoring, and teaching.
	Interdisciplinary collaboration.
	Initiate and coordinate referrals.
Focus on secondary and tertiary prevention.	Manage allocated resources.
	Assure outcomes are met.

assess such factors as health status, functional patterns, coping status, and the home/community environment. This assessment results in a database from which nursing diagnoses are formulated, other resource needs determined, and a teaching plan is designed. Planning with the client and the family occurs through a mutual contracting process that involves goal setting, negotiation of responsibilities for plan implementation, and joint evaluation of outcomes. The primary nurse identifies standards of care, critical pathways, or care maps appropriate to the client situation. Care is delegated to the associate nurse if clients are expected to fall within normal expectations over a time line; however, supervision of the case is maintained by the primary nurse. The main focus is on achieving future outcomes and intervening whenever there are significant variations from the norm, ambiguous outcomes, or unpredictable responses that go beyond expected clinical pathways. The primary nurse coordinates the care experience, assures that clinical outcomes are met, collaborates with multiple disciplines, and manages allocated resources.

The associate nurse remains more present-oriented and primarily focuses on implementation of the plan through direct nursing care activities. Clients should have common, well-defined nursing diagnoses with clearly defined standards of care, protocols, and/or pathways and predictable outcomes. To contribute data for reformulation of the nursing diagnoses and a revision of the plan of care, the associate nurse must be highly competent in the assessment of commonly occurring changes in physiological and psychological status, as well as the home environment. The associate nurse works with the client and family, implements and modifies the teaching plan, and is well grounded in secondary and tertiary prevention concepts in order to quickly detect signs and symptoms of potential problems and prevent complications from existing health problems.

The advanced practice nurse (APN) in a managed care environment develops research-based care paths, protocols, and standards, manages large volumes of aggregate information, provides consultation on highly complex client situations, and focuses on the care of clients as they move across a continuum of health care services. This clinician needs to manage the care of groups using fixed dollars and yet achieve high quality clinical outcomes. The use of a team approach in which the APN focuses on population outcomes, the primary nurse is the individual/family case manager, and the associate nurse provides most of the direct skilled nursing care, allows each nurse's knowledge and skills to be used in a cost-effective manner. For example, advanced practice nurses will be in great demand if they can demonstrate to payers and administrators of managed care systems that they can provide cost-effective care to a group of clients with congestive heart failure by the use of a team of home care nurses who can do intensive teaching on health maintenance and self-monitoring. The APN will need to provide group outcome data demonstrating a decrease in visits to the emergency room, hospital readmissions and costly interventions, and an increase in client satisfaction.

Although there are limited studies on the cost of using a differentiated practice model in acute care or home care, Sioux Valley Hospital, a Healing Web group project site for over six years, has demonstrated significant cost savings.

> The implementation of differentiated practice along with shared governance and case management in an extensive six-year process has resulted in decreased lengths of stay, decreased intensive care days, decreased numbers of readmissions, and decreased numbers of inpatient days. During one evaluation of a six-month test period for 35 complex patients, the cost savings for this institution totaled $552,666. . . . The guiding principle used for the implementation and continued refinement of this care delivery model was to place the highest quality-lowest cost provider next to the patient, based on the patient's individual needs at any particular stage of his or her illness or event. (AACN, 1995 pp. 7–8)

SUGGESTED HOME CARE CONTENT FOR ADN AND BSN CURRICULA

For nurses from a variety of educational programs to develop competencies necessary for effective home health nursing practice, curricula must be reexamined and redesigned. If the vast majority of nurses will soon be practicing in nonacute care settings, nursing educators must accomplish major curriculum revisions. Home care and community-based practice is not hospital care in another setting. The acute care setting generally provides more opportunities for immediate assistance and supervision; more independent judgment is needed to practice in the home setting. The client has control over the environment in which the care is provided, and the context of the client's family, home, and community environment becomes crucial in establishing an ongoing therapeutic relationship.

Table 8–3 lists suggested content for associate and baccalaureate nursing programs providing students with the theory base needed for

Table 8–3
Suggested Home Care Content for
ADN and BSN Curricula

Associate Degree Nursing Programs

Coping with chronic illness.
Rehabilitation.
Continuum of health services.
Family (dynamics, as the unit of service, assessment, and coping).
Effect of attitudes, beliefs, values on health.
Self-care and caregiver education.
Home assessment and modification.
Family/client teaching.
Supervision and delegation of client care.
Levels of prevention.
Case finding.
Community resources.
Health team collaboration.
Assessment of family caregiver capabilities.
Home care clinical laboratory experience.

Additional Content for Baccalaureate Nursing Programs

Epidemiology.
Statistics.
Family contracting.
Community assessment.
Public health science.
Environmental health.
Negotiation.
Health care economics and financing.
Management of allocated resources.
Politics and policy development.
Family systems theory.
Determinants of health.
Health promotion and protection.
Interdisciplinary collaboration.
Design and evaluation of teaching/self-monitoring plans.
Case management.
Quality assurance.
Nursing information systems.

beginning-level practice in home settings. Associate degree educators need to reassess the current focus on the hospital as the primary clinical learning laboratory. As the shift from hospital to home progresses, there is an increasing need for ADN graduates to become more fully integrated into community-based care. Clinical laboratory experiences of the future should include provision of experiences in home care, ambulatory care settings, long-term care, and other less structured community settings so that students have more opportunities to experiment with creative approaches to client health care needs and to develop critical thinking skills. Tagliareni and Murray (1995) stress the need for associate degree nurse educators to offer community-based clinical experiences in which students can work with clients over an extended period to ". . . understand collaboration, to challenge assumptions, and to utilize reflective, inquiry methods of decision making" (p. 370).

SUMMARY

Nursing education curricula must be designed to meet changing societal needs, as well as changes in the approach to health care financing and delivery. To utilize and value the knowledge and skills of all nurses, home care could be delivered through a coordinated approach using the Healing Web Model of differentiated practice. Selected competencies for the associate, primary, and advanced practice roles were presented and curricular revisions incorporating home care content were suggested. Although many nurses will still practice in acute high-tech institutes, the majority of nursing care will be delivered in long-term care facilities and community settings. A delineation of roles and a restructuring of curricula will facilitate a transition from a primary focus on provision of acute episodic care to community-based care for ambulatory populations and chronically ill clients in home and long-term care settings.

REFERENCES

American Association of Colleges of Nursing. (1995). *A model for differentiated nursing practice*. Washington, DC: Author.

Hanner, M. B. (1985). Associate and baccalaureate degree preparation for future clinical practice in home health care. *Journal of the New York State Nurses Association, 16*, 31–37.

Larson, J. (1992). The healing web: A transformative model for nursing. *Nursing & Health Care, 13,* 246–252.

Larson, J., Johnson, S., Holmes, P. K., Leuning, C., & Schuller, L. (1995). The healing web: Curriculum changes to support differentiated practice roles in the community. In P. Bayles & J. Parks-Doyle (Eds.), *The web of inclusion: Faculty helping faculty* (pp. 123–132). New York: National League for Nursing Press.

Tagliareni, M. E., & Murray, J. P. (1995). Community-focused experiences in the ADN curriculum. *Journal of Nursing Education, 34,* 366–371.

9

A Differentiated Practice Model

How Connecting with a City Health Department
Provides Unique Learning Experiences

June Larson
Carol Stuart
Susan Johnson

HISTORY OF THE HEALING WEB

Our story shows how a public associate degree nursing program and a private baccalaureate nursing program joined with a health care system and a city health department to provide new learning experiences for students. Looking back to the process that nourished such partnerships is important. As such, the Healing Web is a model for the reconciliation and transformation of nursing (Bunkers et al., 1992; Larson et al., 1992). Since 1990, the leadership and nursing faculty and staff from the University of South Dakota (USD), Augustana College, and Sioux Valley Hospital have worked on a collaborative model that facilitates change in both education and practice. In 1992, the creation of the Healing Web Institute formalized this partnership. The Web expanded in 1993 as the National Healing Web Partners formed, bringing in Web groups from Montana, Utah, Minnesota, and Wisconsin. Trust has been an essential element of the relationships in this partnership. Trust is integral to the formation of a collective purpose.

Key Concepts of the Healing Web

Margaret Newman's theory, "Health as Expanding Consciousness," and Native American culture and traditions have had an impact on the philosophy and conceptual framework of the Healing Web Model. The Healing Web core group has embraced Native American beliefs concerning the healing powers of the web. The web, associated with spinning and weaving, is believed to be an effort in creative transformation and part of a healing discipline. To the Healing Web core group, the metaphor of the WEB seemed fitting for our work (Figure 9–1). The

**Figure 9–1
The Healing Web**

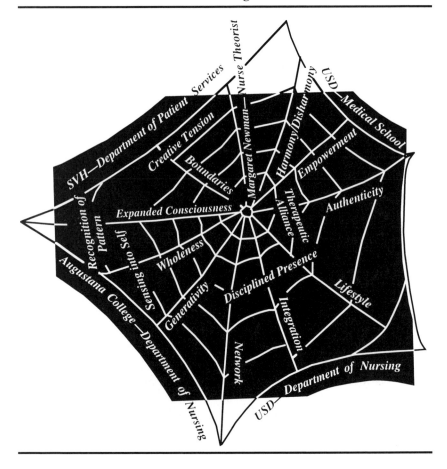

Figure 9–2
Acronym for the Healing Web

Harmony
Empowerment
Authenticity
Lifestyle
Integration
Network
Generativity
Wholeness
Expanded Consciousness
Boundaries

---

bridge line in the Healing Web Model is nurse theorist Margaret Newman. The radial lines are the concepts used in developing curriculum and the source for the acronym HEALING WEB (Figure 9–2; Bunkers et al., 1992).

Nursing: The Past and the Future

In the Healing Web Model, the past is depicted by a stepladder (Figure 9–3), representing a hierarchical structure where the nurse gains

Figure 9–3
Nursing Hierarchical Structure

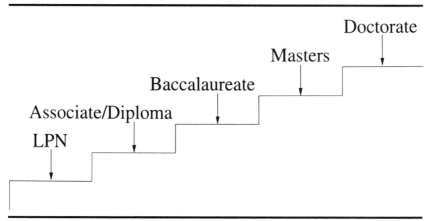

Figure 9–4
The Whole of Nursing

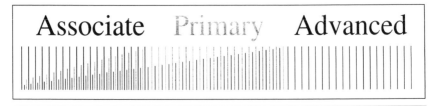

Note: From Larson et al., 1992. Reprinted by permission of author.

importance and power with education and/or each move up the ladder. The Healing Web Model, the future, is depicted by a continuum that represents unity and connectedness (Figure 9–4; Larson et al., 1992). In this "whole" of nursing, no nurse commands higher esteem than another. The role of each nurse is specifically defined, and the value and worth of expertise in each role is equal although the time orientation, complexity of function, and emphasis in practice will differ. The unique contributions of each role and the diversity of role relationships are valued. As the nurse moves along the continuum, the complexity of function and emphasis in practice change, yet the value of each individual's role is viewed as equal to others. Each nurse is a part of the whole of nursing. Collaborative practice utilizing all roles is the whole of nursing practice. Within the framework of the Healing Web Model, through mutual valuing, integration, and collaboration, nurses begin to relate in a new and cooperative way. In this model, students from the University of South Dakota Associate of Arts nursing program and students from the Augustana College baccalaureate nursing program began working in the complementary roles of associate and primary nurse to provide care to clients on a clinical unit within Sioux Valley Hospital's differentiated practice model. This collaborative effort was designed to facilitate educational preparation for both newly emerging practice roles and future nursing practice roles. Within this acute care setting, the associate nurse provides comfort and physiological stabilization and the baccalaureate nurse provides continuity of care and a timely prepared discharge (Pitts-Wilhelm, Nicolai, & Koerner, 1991). This acute care clinical learning experience has demonstrated that "nursing is relational," a belief central to the work of the Healing Web.

Council Process

The Healing Web core group uses council process as a means of communication. This process, a Native American tradition, involves a focused state of listening. There are three simple rules: Speak honestly. Be brief. Listen from the heart. The "talking stick" is passed in the direction of the sun. Each person speaks in turn when he or she is handed the talking stick and only while holding it. It is important not to speak out of turn. This helps to focus attention on listening rather than speaking. Trust is built with focused listening. It is in the silence that much is understood.

Curriculum Revision and the Move to Community

Curriculum revision with clinical learning experiences in the community has taken place concurrently with our work in developing the Healing Web Model. In response to society's evolving health care needs, we felt a need to move to community, with an emphasis on disease prevention and health promotion. Within this curriculum, communities are seen as an essential and permanent part of the lived human experience; community is caring for "Person" (each individual) in the lived environment.

Community as Part of the "Lived Human Experience"

Faculty spent considerable time discussing the role of associate degree graduates in the community. We have chosen to provide learning experiences of caring for Person in the lived environment, rather than to provide learning experiences of caring for the community. In choosing community clinical experiences, we sought experiences that provide the opportunity to work with culturally diverse persons and with vulnerable persons, to collaborate with other health team members, and to implement health promotion and disease prevention.

Role Differentiation in Community We are in the process of identifying role differentiation in the community. At USD, we have begun to identify what we believe the role of the AD graduates to be and the relationship to graduates from other educational backgrounds. The associate role includes promotion of health, prevention of health problems (includes education), identification of specific interventions for disease, rehabilitation, evaluation of the plan of care, and contribution to research.

Nursing skills needed in the community include expert assessment skills, advocate for Person, the empowerment of Person to meet his or her own needs and gain control of his or her own life; partner with Person, sharing the skills of decision making, priority setting, and health teaching.

Multidisciplinary Clinic

The work of the Healing Web is evolving and has included community experiences with a Visiting Nurse's Association (Larson et al., 1995) and currently a multidisciplinary acute care clinic supported by outside governmental funding. In planning for a differentiated practice clinical experience in the acute care clinic, key persons from the involved institutions and agencies met and explored the feasibility and possibilities of such a project. Representatives from Augustana College, the University of South Dakota, Sioux Valley Hospital, Sioux River Valley Community Health Center, and the South Dakota Department of Health were present. Attitudes gradually moved from questioning and skepticism to a strong commitment to the project. Open communication and trusting relationships, which were the hallmark of the original project as well as these early discussions, remain essential to the planning and implementation of ongoing activities in the community. All the participants, including the students, needed to accept the reality that we had more questions than answers and that we were doing something new and unique. We learned to live with this ambiguity and had to be willing to let the project evolve. Certainly, our work with differentiated practice in the community can be viewed as "an evolving pattern of the whole" (Newman, 1986). We are comfortable with "throwing the road out before us." We believe that our nursing practice will inform us about the specific roles in the community that make up the whole of nursing.

A Lived Experience in the Community Health Center

One placement to which students have been assigned is a collaborative, multidisciplinary clinic, a setting that values culture, gender, and life experiences to promote a healing perspective. A focus of this Healing Web community project was to determine if (and how) the roles of the associate and baccalaureate degree nurses are differentiated in the community setting. Another exciting and unique facet of the community clinical experience was to explore and identify the emerging roles of the master's and doctoral prepared nurses in the community setting. Four second-year students from the University of South Dakota Associate Degree Program participated in the project for 6 weeks during the fall semester and another 4 weeks during the spring semester. At the same time, six students from the Augustana College Baccalaureate Program also participated in clinical learning experiences, which facilitated having the same students together in the community setting for a total of 10 weeks during the academic school year.

The USD associate students were assigned to partner with either the clinic nurse who worked most directly with the primary care provider or the registered nurse in the Women, Infants, and Children (WIC) office, certifying or counseling clients. The Augustana College baccalaureate students talked to patients in the waiting room at the clinic, prepared charts with the desk nurse, triaged patients, responded to phone calls, and worked with clinic staff organizing and implementing an immunization program. In the WIC office, the baccalaureate students partnered with the RN in the Baby Care Program or the RN who had management responsibilities.

Although the students assigned to the clinic interacted with patients at different phases of their visit, it was feasible to communication with each other about the patients as needed. Two student partners had a unique opportunity to collaborate about the status of a patient with the potential of impacting care beyond the reason that prompted the current visit. The patient came to the clinic with what appeared to be a "minor injury." As her story unfolded, it became apparent that there was real cause for concern about her involvement in an abusive relationship. This encounter enabled the students to learn from each other and to appreciate different perspectives.

There were ongoing opportunities to identify and understand the influence of cultural and socioeconomic values and attitudes on daily living practices and health. Faculty, staff, and students gained insight into the lived experiences of the clients' lives as well as of each other's.

Shared Learning through Clinical Conferences Because the community setting requires that nurses function more independently and because students were assigned to different responsibilities and to different geographic locations, the postconferences were critical in bringing all pieces together in a shared learning experience. It was a time for reflecting on issues or experiences. In the interaction, master's and doctoral prepared nurses had the opportunity to frame and pose questions meant to expand emotional and cognitive processes. To open our minds to the potential of what *can be,* brain teasers were used to jar our brains out of their cognitive ruts and challenge our thought processes. We have learned how a "mind-set" or habit can block our communication or perhaps block our creativity. We realized the need to break out of our old patterns and the "business-as-usual" mentality.

Whether the conference was an informal time of sharing or a more structured process, it modeled the caring and mutual valuing of each person. The dynamics could be described as relational based on participating in the experiences of each other and building relationships through the telling and hearing of each person's story. In this way, we came to understand another person's lived experience, and we became connected to each other. No participant will ever be quite the same again.

STORY TELLING

The stories of the clients were incredible. There were the recently immigrated parents who spoke very little English who came to the clinic to have their child's immunization record evaluated. They kept the appointment to bring the health records from their country of origin, even though the child was in school. The incredible part is that the parents were not sure where the school was. All they knew was that a big yellow bus picked their child up in the morning and brought him back again in the afternoon. Where he was during the day was a mystery to them.

A middle-aged woman with a blood pressure of 200/120 had medication prescribed. On subsequent visits, she explained how her dog ate the pills or how she accidentally spilled the bottle of her medication down the drain. Investigation revealed she had never purchased the medication because she couldn't afford it and was too embarrassed to admit this. She hadn't realized the clinic could help her.

These are only two of the threads pulled from the rich tapestry of life, which is woven each day in this community setting, that helped to facilitate the students' recognition and understanding of lived experiences.

Evaluation after the First Year

Joint evaluation of students and their staff partners revealed positive experiences even though the "if" and "how" of differentiation were not readily apparent because a differentiated practice model is not currently in place at the community clinic. The learning objectives of each educational program had been shared among all students and staff at the beginning of the experience. It was primarily through these objectives that differentiation of the associate and baccalaureate roles could be demonstrated. Differentiation of roles by educational preparation remains a focus of the Healing Web community project as we plan experiences for the second year.

The power contribution of this experience in the lives of faculty, students, and staff lies in changed ideas, attitudes, and feelings. In partnership with the clients and with each other, we learned to understand and value lived experiences.

In the journaling process, one student shared this insight: "I went to the clinic with a predetermined attitude about "those people" who come to a federally funded free clinic. I spent time getting to know these people. I left feeling tremendously changed. I realized "those" people are like me and could be me if my life's circumstances changed. And that wouldn't take much!"

This healing community within the Healing Web is socializing the students to value diversity and the unique contributions of each Person. Relationships that result in mutual understanding, valuing, and respect will facilitate healing.

REFERENCES

Bunkers, S. with Brendiro, M., Holmes, P. K., Howell, J., Johnson, S., Koemer, J., Larson, J., Nelson, J., & Weaver, R. (1992). "The healing web: A transformative model for nursing. *Nursing and Health Care, 13*(1), 69–73.

Larson, J. with Auterman, M., Brendiro, M., Bunkers, L., Bunkers, S., Cranston, V., Dore-Paulson, C., Holmes, P. K., Howell, J., Johnson, S., Karpiuk, K., Koemer, J., Nelson, J., Nelson, M., & Weaver, R. (1992). "The healing web: A transformative model for nursing. Part II. *Nursing and Health Care, 13*(5), 246–252.

Larson, J. (1995). The healing web: Curriculum changes to support differentiated practice roles in the community. In *The Web of inclusion: Faculty helping faculty.* (Publication #14-2682). New York: National League for Nursing Press.

Newman, M. (1986). *Health as expanding consciousness.* St. Louis: Mosby.

Pitts-Wilhelm, P., Nicolai, C., & Koerner, J. (1991). Differentiating nursing practice to improve service outcomes. *Nursing Management, 22*(12), 22–25.

10

Creating a Community-Based Interdisciplinary Collaborative Practice Model within a Mobile Nurse-Managed Health Center

Evelyn Atchison
Charlene Connolly

The Division of Health Technologies, Northern Virginia Community College (NVCC) has recognized the need to be proactive in redefining the role of nursing and allied health pracitioners at the associate degree level, transforming curricula to meet the changing demands of health care and being proactive in establishing complementary pathways within community-based health care services. The division enrolls approximately 1,200 students each academic year, offering eight associate degree programs: Nursing, Dental Hygiene, Emergency Medical Technology, Health Information Technology, Medical Laboratory Technology, Physical Therapist Assisting, Radiography, and Respiratory Therapy. In addition, several certificate programs ranging from entry level to postassociate degree are available.

In 1994, an assessment of NVCC's nursing and allied health students' attitudes toward providing community-based health services indicated a trend across all disciplines: While students generally identified the importance of providing community-based services, the majority of students attached a high value only to those roles associated with acute care. This was a disturbing finding; the need to enhance nursing and allied health students' commitment to community-based care and public service became critically evident to us.

In addition, faculty sought a way to not only better define the roles of the associate degree nurse, but to enhance that functioning through the development of collaborative, inclusion-rich, community-based practice experiences. Inquiry was based on the premise that if nursing is to meet the demands of a rapidly changing health care system in which there are expanding and diverse health care settings, demands for cost containment, and the need to increase access to quality care, a delivery model must be developed that differentiates scopes of job responsibility on the basis of education, competence, and experience.

Due to the anticipated changes in health care, differentiated nursing practice that includes all levels of nursing education is beginning to be nationally implemented in varied community-based health care delivery settings. Viewed as a collaborative practice model, differentiated nursing practice can be defined as "the practice of structuring nursing roles on the basis of education, experience and practice," (Boston, 1990). Because these differentiated nursing models do not focus on interdisciplinary practice, NVCC nursing and allied health faculty expanded this concept creating a *collaborative* differentiated practice framework.

The vision of a practice environment that developed at NVCC was one in which the associate degree nursing student would become an integral component of differentiated practice teams. These teams would be operating under a faculty practice model with leadership generated by nursing faculty and professional staff consisting of advanced practice professionals: physicians, nurse practitioners, and physician assistants. These teams would also be working within an interdisciplinary framework with three different levels of nursing students, as well as allied health students and nursing faculty to provide a broad scope of primary health care and health promotion screenings and services in community-based settings in the northern Virginia region.

The defined roles of the three levels of nursing students, associate (ADN), baccalaureate (BSN), and master's degree (MSN), relate to the function that each performs in providing care to the client and the role each holds according to the educational background of the student. For example, the ADN student is prepared to provide nursing care to clients who have uncomplicated, commonly defined conditions. The role differentiation of the ADN student is that of being assistive to other health care providers when clients have complicated and less defined conditions. In contrast, the BSN student is prepared to provide nursing care to clients who have unusual or unpredictable conditions. The role differentiation is that of being fully responsible for the client's care in collaboration with other health care providers. The MSN student functions in a much broader scope of practice compared with the BSN student in that the nursing care provided is more comprehensive. The MSN student's role is to lead the interdisciplinary team, and coordination of care is a major responsibility.

MOBILE NURSE-MANAGED HEALTH CENTER

In response to this vision, the Division of Health Technologies was successful in receiving grant funding from the Corporation for National Service, Learn and Serve America: Higher Education, in partnership with other institutions of higher education, local community agencies, county health departments, and other public and private nonprofit agencies. This funding supports the implementation of a community-based clinical practice, a *Mobile Nurse-Managed Health Center Program (MNMHC)*.

The purpose of the MNMHC is to develop a demonstration model of community-based clinical practice, incorporating service-learning, differentiated practice, and caring, as a structured part of nursing and allied health curricula. As an outreach effort focusing on community, cultural, physical, and civic/social needs, NVCC nursing and allied health students provide free primary health care services to special populations in the northern Virginia area. Each academic year, 300 nursing and allied health students provide primary health care and health promotion services to approximately 1,500 individuals at over 25 community-based sites.

The outcomes of the MNMHC address three impacts: community (client), participant (student), and institutional (organization/agencies).

Community Impact Outcomes

Develop self-care skills and attitudes.

Utilize appropriate community services to meet health care needs.

Assume primary responsibility for health care decisions.

Participant Impact Outcomes

Develop an appreciation for community service.

Explore community-based careers.

Provide competent health care services to diverse populations based on the caring model.

Strengthen collaborative relationships based on collaborative differentiated practice.

Institutional Impact Outcomes

Develop community-based curricula.

Strengthen community partnerships to sustain the MNMHC.

Increase NVCC's recognition of service-learning.

Improve inclusion, collaboration, and role differentiation among regional nursing and allied health programs.

To accomplish the outcomes associated with the MNMHC project, major curricular changes have taken place, incorporating service-learning, differentiated practice, and caring experiences through the implementation of the Mobile Nurse-Managed Health Center. Figure 10–1 illustrates the revision from the former Nursing Curriculum to the current Nursing Curriculum noting the changes in the practice environment, emphasis on interdisciplinary teams, and collaborative differentiated practice. These changes have resulted in significant differences in faculty and student roles and responsibilities, focus of care, and closer connections with an increased understanding of the health needs of our communities.

SERVICE-LEARNING

The blending of academic study and community service is an integral aspect of the MNMHC. Stuctured service-learning experiences serve as a basis for weekly community-based clinical rotations that meet the following objectives: (1) identify individual risk-factors, (2) promote positive health habits, (3) motivate individuals to set healthier lifestyle goals, (4) provide primary care services, and (5) initiate appropriate referrals and follow-up.

The MNMHC is managed by two full-time faculty who are family nurse pracitioners and staffed by a medical director, a physician assistant, part-time nurse pracitioners and a van coordinator who are considered part of the interdisciplinary team along with the faculty and students. The plan for collaborative inclusion has been designed so that each time the MNMHC is operational, a core of five ADN, two BSN, and one MSN nursing students and two allied health students representing the

Figure 10–1
Comparison of Former and Current Nursing Curriculum

Former Nursing Curriculum	Current Nursing Curriculum
1. Faculty-designed clinical practicum.	1. Student-designed clinical practicum.
2. Community service activities are voluntary with no follow-up.	2. Community service activities are a structured part of the Reflective Educational Curriculum framework.
3. Clinical rotations include community-based service, observational only.	3. Primary care is delivered; interactive clinical rotations occur as part of the MNMHC.
4. Clinical practicums are hospital controlled.	4. Clinical practicums are client/population controlled.
5. Focus is on leadership and management in the hospital setting.	5. Focus is on change agents identifying unmet community needs and ways to positively influence meeting those needs.
6. Students focus on costs and quality.	6. Students focus on accessing quality care for clients through collaborative practice.
7. Nursing practice is based on Modified Primary Functional Care Delivery Model.	7. Nursing practice using an interdisciplinary team based on differentiated practice and caring model.
8. Students focus on individual clients and their community, cultural, and social needs, and how they affect the patient.	8. Students focus on the client's community, cultural, and social needs and relate unmet needs as causative agents to the disease processes.
9. Students focus on the acute or episodic aspects of illness.	9. Students focus on assessment and health promotion and disease prevention.

disciplines of Dental Hygiene, Emergency Medical Services, Medical Laboratory Technology, Radiography, Respiratory Therapy, Medical Office Management, and/or Physical Therapist Assisting as appropriate, are assigned to the unit. A nursing faculty from the community college is assigned direct clinical instruction for this practicum. Nursing faculty have full authority and responsibility for student learning and safety while they are assigned to the MNMHC.

Each ADN student participates in 64 hours of primary health care services during a four-week community-based practicum. BSN and MSN nursing students are assigned to the mobile unit for longer periods. Health care services are offered four days per week at more than 25 different community-based sites. Health assessment, screenings, client education, and chronic disease monitoring are the major services provided. Clients are given access to primary and preventive health care services on a weekly basis, allowing for return visits. Clients are provided with referral and action plans to better understand how to become more self-sufficient in obtaining health care resources for themselves and their families.

A major component of this experience is the emphasis on the students' civic/social responsibility and commitment to community-based service. The structured service-learning experiences include exposure to specific populations. The ADN and BSN students are given the opportunities to assess, teach, monitor, interview, make referrals, and write client action plans. All students participating in service-learning activities not only provide direct community service, but also learn about the context in which the service is provided, and understand the connection between the service and their academic course work. Students representing all levels are assigned special responsibilities related to client care and health problems that include assessment of the problem, analysis of the problem, development of goals and objectives to respond to the problem, response to the problem, and finally evaluation of the results from actions taken.

Faculty supervise all aspects of the students' service experiences. They hold pre- and postconferences daily to facilitate students' reflection on the experiences as a whole and on individual client problems. These reflections are shared among all students in the group and enable them to collectively use critical thinking skills to resolve immediate threats to an individual's or the community's health and welfare. Students write a paper on the service experience according to structured guidelines. Capacity building activities are included that focus on educating both students and faculty in health education techniques and theories associated with behavior changes such as those dealing with self-efficacy. Specific strategies are implemented to assist the students to effect positive behavior change in their clients. Additionally, students are in-serviced in regard to case management, coordination of care, referrals to community resources, home care services, and the concepts of managed care. These aspects of training have been incorporated into the curriculum and are identified by specific competencies and objectives. Additional video and computer resources related to community-based care and health promotion and education are available for students' use.

Students become familiar with the concepts of language-appropriate health information and education resources. Students utilize their knowledge of cultural orientations of individuals when planning care for clients representing diverse population groups.

As an identified clinical practicum, the value of the MNMHC community-based experience becomes heightened. Students identify with the positive aspects of providing care to underserved populations and recognize the paradigm shift in the provision of health care services to the community setting.

COLLABORATIVE DIFFERENTIATED PRACTICE

Collaborative relationships among nurses and other health care providers of the MNMHC are based on mutual valuing in which each person's expertise is recognized and respected. The model is implemented by matching each health care provider's different and unique capabilities with the client's different and unique health care needs. The goal is to define the role of each provider so that each provider contributes in some way to the client's care (AACN-AONE, 1995).

An important component of the process of creating a collaborative differentiated practice model is the need for inclusion of educators from each discipline at all program levels in the planning process. We have found that inclusion of all allied health educators and nursing educators, as well as educators from advanced practice, physician assistant, and medical schools, especially those in primary care, are essential for success. Frequent meetings of these educators are necessary to reach agreement on each program's learning objectives and the choice of appropriate practice sites that will enhance differentiated practice roles and levels. This sharing process creates an environment that fosters caring relationships among team members and brings about cost-effective and quality client care.

Implementation of a collaborative model such as differentiation of practice roles does not require major changes to the discipline curricula. Instead, a willingness among all levels of educators in each discipline to incorporate concepts of collaboration into practice can in itself serve as an example of collaboration.

A specific student outcome for the MNMHC is to strengthen collaborative relationships. Therefore we chose to approach our demonstration project through a collaborative differentiated practice model focusing on an interdisciplinary team concept. For our purposes, role differentiation among allied health and nursing students at the associate degree level was structured horizontally and three levels of nursing students were structured vertically.

Consequently, implementation of role differentiation of nursing and allied health students at the associate degree level is structured according to specific discipline competencies at the same educational level. Currently, NVCC nursing, respiratory therapy, dental hygiene, and medical laboratory students are actively involved in the MNMHC program. Role differentiation among associate (ADN), baccalaureate (BSN), and master's degree (MSN) nursing students is structured according to specific education levels and competencies within the same discipline.

INTERDISCIPLINARY TEAMS

Implementing an interdisciplinary team concept is achieved through the inclusion of staff and students from each nursing and allied health discipline and level. College faculty are also a part of the team and are necessary for appropriate supervision of student performance. All levels of disciplines of health care providers in the MNMHC program are expected to meet regularly and share responsibilities for the program's development and maintenance. Some of the discussion involves planning the flow of services, determining supply and equipment needs of the program, and discussing services and client/population needs. The development of roles for each health care provider and/or student is also the responsibility of the team. Roles are defined according to the current literature on differentiation and applied to student competencies and outcomes for learning. According to Bloomer (1983), "The education of health care professionals should emphasize a strong sense of professional identity and clarity regarding roles, functions and responsibilities entrusted to that professional in various practice settings." Without the necessary identity and clarity of professional roles among all health care providers, there will be disharmony and, less quality of health care services, and cost-containment effort will suffer.

For example, allied health students in the respiratory program are responsible for completing an in-depth assessment of the client's respiratory system; the medical laboratory students are responsible for obtaining blood and other specimens as determined by the physician, physician assistant, or the nurse practitioner; and dental hygiene students complete oral assessments including cancer screenings. Plans exist for inclusion of all seven allied health program students, including medical office management students, who will maintain client records and assist with clinic office responsibilities.

ADN nursing students, serving as the critical core of the MNMHC, are responsible for completing the intake interview and the client's history form. Determining the chief complaint of the client is the major competency of this activity. During this time, initial vital signs can be obtained and recorded by the ADN student. The ADN student, along with faculty guidance, determines appropriate access for primary care services to the nurse practitioner, physician assistant, medical director, or the BSN student for patient teaching or referrals.

The BSN student is usually responsible for teaching the client and often makes referrals to other health care providers and/or agencies. Follow-up is the responsibility of either the ADN or BSN student. The MSN student completes a health assessment of the client under the nurse practitioner's or physician's supervision and often assists with coordination of client care given by the ADN and BSN students.

CARING MODEL

Another component of the collaborative differentiated practice model is application of the caring model. Caring is an essential component to strengthening collaborative relationships. Valuing and respecting the expertise of each health care provider is a form of caring. By demonstrating caring attitudes and behaviors toward members of the interdisciplinary team, students are helped to transfer human caring from self and the team to the client. Inclusion is a challenge that does not happen automatically. Concepts such as leadership, conflict management and delegation of tasks among the team are applied to the setting by the faculty to demonstrate to students the legal and ethical parameters of the team concept. Caring relationships among team members are essential in developing effective working relationships both across and within disciplines.

CONCLUSION

Building capacity through collaboration has been a hallmark of the Division of Health Technologies at Northern Virginia Community College. Division programs are recognized as a major contributor to the skilled health profession's labor pool, orchestrating a vital leadership role in nursing and allied health education in the region. In fact, 85 percent of the health care workforce in northern Virginia are graduates of the college; each year's graduating class provides care for over 500,000 individuals.

Through the implementation of programs such as the Mobile Nurse-Managed Health Center, it becomes evident that strong leadership for change exists at the community college. Community college nursing and allied health faculty are eager to advocate for inclusion of other college and university faculty as a strategy to advance health care practice and education. The network, resources, and relationships that NVCC enjoys extend to urban, suburban, and rural communities.

An exciting future awaits the faculty, students, and community members in this region. Through respect and recognition of the value that each nursing and allied health program offers in working together, true collaboration can help every partner reach beyond his or her individual potential. The result has to be a better educated health care workforce able to meet the demands of a changing practice paradigm toward community-based care.

REFERENCES

AACN-AONE Task Force. (1995). A Model for Differentiated Practice. American Association of Colleges of Nursing. 12–13:28–29.

Bloomer, J. S. (1983). Interdisciplinary health care teams: Conflict or collaboration? A review of the literature on working role relations. Unpublished Manuscript, Florida State University.

Boston, C. (1990). Differentiated practice: An introduction." In C. Boston (Ed.), Current issues and perspectives on differentiated practice (pp. 1–3). Chicago: American Organization of Nurse Executives.

Watson, J. (1988). A case-study: Curriculum in transition. In Curriculum revolution: Mandate for change. New York: NLN Press.

SECTION IV

Curriculum Models for Integration of Community Concepts

11

Community Infusion

New Strategies for Teaching the Three Levels of Prevention

Barbara B. Marckx
Janet Z. Denman

During the January 1993 semester break, the entire nursing faculty at Broome Community College met at a retreat center to brainstorm the future direction and goals of the associate degree program. Based on the Pew Health Professions Commission Report (Shugars, O'Neil, & Bader, 1991) and the local trend in health care delivery, an emphasis on community-based care emerged. A commitment was made to modify our program to step into the 21st century where cost containment would drive health care and community settings would replace institutionally based care. A literature search revealed only one article (Davis & McKee-Johnson, 1988) connecting associate degree education and community nursing, but it was enough to get us started.

PILOT PROJECT

Working on a college minigrant, four adjunct instructors, all community health prepared, formed a subcommittee to investigate the introduction of community-based experiences into the program. Hospital discharge planners and home care coordinators from various community agencies were approached. The broad objectives were to expose students to wider opportunities for nurses and to emphasize the importance of patient teaching in preparation for discharge from the hospital. Specific objectives were developed as well as a tool for written completion following the experience. A grid was devised to organize the visits and each senior medical-surgical clinical instructor assigned a student to the community agency/hospital for a one-day observation. The theoretical component for these observations was developed as a 75-minute Community Health class consisting of a role-play scenario, a brief historical view of home care, the concept of community health and case management, the role of the visiting nurse, and a case study. By the time this first phase of community infusion was implemented, the National League for Nursing (1993) had issued a statement that community is the thrust of the future and nurses at all levels need this experience. Their directive confirmed our commitment to provide community-based experiences as preparation for employment as a registered nurse.

The second phase of community infusion involved changes in the senior-level, five-week Pediatric clinical rotation necessitated by significant problems in securing adequate acute care experiences. Again adjunct instructors took the lead and placed students in a variety of community-based settings. To provide meaningful experiences without an instructor's presence, site-specific objectives, databases, and evaluation forms were developed as written assignments. One of the most creative and successful experiences designed was the Pediatric Health Fair (see Chapter 23).

CURRICULUM REVISION

At the present time, our curriculum is undergoing extensive changes in response to demands for primary prevention, enhanced assessment skills, and out-of-hospital or community care. We have selected an eclectic caring philosophy and the structural framework of Gordon's (1982) 11 patterns of human functioning. In this third phase of our infusion project, community concepts form essential components that are woven throughout the curriculum in class and clinical objectives and activities, writing experiences, and nursing skills center activities.

Freshman Level

In the first semester, students are introduced to basic components of community nursing as they study an overview of Gordon's 11 patterns applied to wellness concepts. The first pattern, Health Maintenance, includes the identification and description of the three levels of illness prevention. Also in this pattern, they explore various settings for the delivery of health services and the trend of moving from hospital to community-based health care. The students' initial clinical experience occurs in a senior citizens' center where the focus is basic communication and blood pressure measurement. For many years, students toured the centers, had lunch with the well elderly, and practiced basic communication skills. This year, in collaboration with the community agency, the faculty changed the order of teaching nursing skills to start with vital signs assessment, which enabled the students to do blood pressure screening on their first clinical day at the centers. A simple card was designed to record the reading for the elder, together with recommended schedules for routine checkups for persons over 60, such as physical, dental, and eye exams. The instructors were present to supervise students and role model problem-solving in answering questions and suggesting interventions. This activity was highly valued by the elders who perceived the students as giving something back to the community through blood pressure screening. In reality, the students gained by having numerous opportunities to take blood pressures on healthy elders, in contrast to learning the skill with a single frail nursing home resident. By collaborating with this community agency, both students and elders experienced satisfaction with the activity and student learning was markedly improved.

During the first few weeks of the semester, the students practiced physical assessment and vital signs measurement in the nursing skills lab. The initial clinical rotation for freshmen, midway in the first semester, is four weeks in a skilled nursing home, where they apply assessment skills learned in the lab. In the nursing home, they provide a tertiary level of prevention by practicing rehabilitative nursing care with the frail elderly. By the time the students enter the hospital during the 10th week, they are more proficient in all assessment skills, including vital signs, than students were in prior classes.

The Community Resource Paper (see Figure 11–1), a class assignment in the first semester, is designed to evaluate students' writing skills and introduce each of them to one community agency. Students are instructed to sign up for the agency they choose to research; which ensures variety within the class and avoids burdening the agencies with multiple student contacts. This information-gathering task teaches the student some of the important facts a nurse needs to know about an agency before recommending it to a client. Included in the assignment is a

Figure 11–1
Community Resource Paper

Purpose: To familiarize the student with resources within the community that assist individuals to maintain health.

Directions: Select a community resource person or organization that individuals may contact for the purpose of maintaining their health.

Write a 2–3 page paper, *typed and double spaced*, that includes:

- Name of organization.
- Contact person.
- Age/group that it serves.
- Cost.
- Level of illness prevention provided.
- Pamphlets or handouts provided.
- Address.

- Purpose of organization.
- Meeting time.
- Services provided.
- Advantages of organization.
- Disadvantages.
- You may include your opinion of the person or organization.

Evaluation

Fifty percent of the grade is devoted to content.

Fifty percent of the grade is devoted to writing ability, such as spelling, punctuation, sentence structure, clarity, grammar, style.

Suggestions

Car Seat Loan	Boys and Girls Clubs
Caregivers Support Group	Boating Safety
Dental Services (NYS donated)	Babysitting Safety Classes
Meals-on-Wheels of Western Broome	Pregnancy Education
Breast Feeding Support—LaLeche League	First Aid Education

Community Resource Reference sheet that the student completes and files in a notebook for future reference for all students and faculty.

In the second semester, students begin to study each of Gordon's 11 patterns in depth and focus on concepts of illness. The Community Health class occurs in the Health Maintenance pattern. In preparation, students complete assigned readings and view the film, *Cultural Diversity and Nursing Practice: Improving Client Response to Health Care* (Concept Media, 1993). Since this pattern also includes perioperative nursing and caring for persons with infectious diseases, the contrast between surgical asepsis in the hospital and medical asepsis in the home is an important concept. Clinical placement is primarily in acute care settings, but may also include tertiary prevention in a rehabilitation unit, a head trauma unit, and community-based care at the secondary level for outpatients in ambulatory surgery. A Teaching-Learning Project was designed as an evaluative writing assignment for the application of teaching skills. Students create teaching materials that demonstrate efficient synthesis of clinical information by preparing a one-page sheet or pamphlet for teaching patients about topics from second-semester class content. Whenever possible, students are encouraged to use their materials for actual teaching of patients in the clinical area. Projects have included such topics as "AIDS Prevention," "Infection Control," "Managing Your Chronic Disease: Diabetes."

Senior Level

In the senior year, students are offered community-based experiences during each of their clinical rotations. During the 1995–1996 academic year, we used 37 different placements, either in the community or with hospital-based outpatients. As we expanded the sites, we worked with our county attorney to design contracts appropriate for all the different agencies. Our goal is to have contracts viable for an undetermined length of time, to eliminate the necessity of negotiating annually. Most agencies have accepted this "all-purpose" contract, although a few have requested minor revisions to meet their particular needs. Since an instructor is rarely available during a community experience, the contract limits student practice to assessments and measurement of vital signs. To encourage critical thinking and focus students on specific objectives for the community experience, special report forms were developed. A generic form is used for some experiences, while for others there are required readings (Cookfair, 1996; Rice, 1996) and questions pertaining to a particular clinical site. Questions direct the student to focus on specific roles of the nurse (National League for Nursing, 1990) such as assessment and teaching, under Provider of Care; collaboration with other health care disciplines, under Manager of Care; and values and ethical concerns, under Member of the Discipline. Some questions require a factual answer, whereas others encourage the student to reflect personal or professional judgment.

Pediatrics   Through May 1996, students had separate rotations in pediatrics and obstetrics. In pediatrics, where inpatient acute care is very limited, students spent about half of their 5-week rotations at community sites developed in Phase II of this project. Several students were rotated out each day, prompting concerns about disconnected learning and reduced opportunity for instructor-student contact for teaching and evaluation. Requiring students to attend pre– and postconferences on community experience days has helped to provide more continuity in this rotation. Experiences included are participating in pediatric clinics, day-care facilities, school nurses' offices, and a developmental center; planning age-appropriate games for a hospital Halloween party; and teaching age-appropriate health promotion at elementary school and community fairs.

Obstetrics   We use the pediatric and maternity units at two area hospitals. At one of them, we have been able to negotiate a home visit program. The instructor accompanies one or two students on each visit to a discharged obstetric patient. During home visits, the students assess the postpartum mother and newborn, and evaluate the family's adjustment to the birth of the infant. The home setting is also an ideal opportunity to experience cultural diversity, which can be a unique experience for instructor and student. On one visit, a white instructor accompanied a black Muslim student to the home of a Muslim patient. During this visit, the instructor experienced role reversal as the student guided her through the appropriate behaviors expected in the Muslim culture. Students also spend one day in either a prenatal clinic or in the office of a nurse midwife. The focus in these sites is primary and secondary prevention with assessment and teaching for the antepartal client. Since one of these clinics is associated with a tertiary level obstetric care facility, students may experience clients with serious and unusual problems as well as those with the common discomforts of a normal pregnancy. During the maternity rotation, all students are required to visit one or two community-based agencies or classes such as Planned Parenthood, Women, Infants, and Children, Childbirth Education, or Lamaze classes. Information about the site is recorded on a report form and shared among the group during clinical conference.

Medical–Surgical   Each student is rotated off an acute-care unit to two community-based sites, which include chemotherapy clinics, breast clinics, and home visits through Hospice or a home-care agency. Their focus is all three levels of prevention. In the clinics, they participate in patient teaching concerning side effects of chemotherapy, psychological responses, and breast self-exams. Observations include administration of chemotherapy, mammography and various types of breast biopsies. Home visits emphasize the importance of physical assessment skills, critical thinking for independent clinical decision making, environmental assessment and communication techniques for facilitating an effective nurse-client relationship. During the visit and while completing the Home Visit Report, the student is challenged to integrate content from general education courses in psychology and sociology, and to apply this knowledge through assessment of the family environment including its values and culture. Witnessing the impact of terminal illness on family caregivers is a memorable experience that enhances the students' skills in preparing families and patients for expectations following hospital discharge.

Nursing Home–Management   Students are assigned to a skilled nursing or a special dementia unit in a nursing home where the focus is geriatric care and management skills. The rotation was patterned after the experience of the Kellogg Nursing Home Partnership project (Waters, 1991) of which the department was a participant. For the community health segment, each student attends a selected support group and makes a report during clinical conference. As a group, the students plan and conduct a health fair for well elders in a senior citizen residence, addressing all three levels of prevention. Participants make the rounds of stations featuring topics such as "Blood Pressure Screening," "Flu Shots, Nutrition Education," "Skin and Visual Changes with Aging," "Daily Foot Care," "Signs and Symptoms of Infection," "Lifestyle Changes," "Medications: Prescription and Over-the-Counter," "Home Safety," "Myths of Aging," "Are you Blue?" (questionnaire), "What You Need to Know before You Have Surgery," "Questions to Ask Your Doctor," and "How to Be an Informed Patient." Students discover firsthand the importance of thorough preparation as well as the value of critical thinking, prudence, and tact in answering the elders' questions.

Psychiatric–Substance Abuse   During this rotation, students are assigned for 2 or 3 days to a drug detoxification or a 28-day drug rehabilitation unit. The remaining days are spent on a psychiatric unit in a general hospital. Each student visits two community sites, which include a social club and day treatment program for persons with mental illness, the alcohol crisis center, an Alcoholics' Anonymous meeting, and a home visit with the geriatric mobile team or with a community mental health nurse. At the social club, students work alongside members with chronic and persistent mental illness doing tasks such as mopping floors, boning chickens, or working in the secretarial unit as a form of tertiary prevention. Questions on the report form direct the students to assess behavior

of persons with mental illness while challenging stereotypical perceptions of the chronically mentally ill. Consistent with our caring philosophy, the report focuses on values and ethical issues and how these affect
nursing practice. The opportunity to experience a community agency
from the consumer's point of view demonstrates how empowerment enhances an individual's ability to function effectively in a social or work
environment. Students are asked to reflect on how, as future managers or
teachers, they could utilize these concepts in their nursing practice.

During the home visit with the geriatric mobile team, students accompany a psychiatric nurse or social worker who is providing secondary
prevention crisis intervention for elders who have been referred by family or acquaintances because of problematic behavior. One visit was initiated by the air traffic controllers from the nearby airport who were
being harassed by an elderly woman who believed the planes were pur-
posely buzzing her house. Following the visit, students share their assessments with the professional and collaborate in the decision making for
case management of the elder.

Students who spend a day with a community mental health nurse visit
developmentally disabled adults and children in private and group homes
and a sheltered workshop. The focus of the visits vary and can include
all three levels of prevention. They frequently report on the teaching
focus of the visit, including medications and physical symptoms management. At one of the visits, the student and nurse provided information
about sterilization to a retarded adolescent and her family, and discussed
the legal and ethical aspects of individual rights, informed consent, and
parental responsibilities.

Intensive Care Unit–Cardiac Care Unit   The ICU/CCU rotation has
been the most challenging area in which to provide a meaningful community experience that justifies removing students from units with rich
hands-on skill opportunities. Visiting a person for home care management of insulin administration and diabetic foot care seemed inappropriate as a replacement for inserting nasogastric tubes or suctioning the
tracheostomy of a ventilator-dependent patient in ICU. The prospect of
increased numbers of students in a clinical group prompted us to think
creatively for community experiences for this rotation. Four ambulance
companies were contacted about the possibility of student experiences
and all enthusiastically welcomed us as participants in their Professional
Ride-Along programs. Students complete a simple waiver form provided
by the company and are scheduled for a six-hour block of time. We

anticipated they would be fascinated by the primary and secondary prevention prehospital management of acute trauma, but found the more common and most meaningful experiences are witnessing the deplorable conditions in many of the homes to which the ambulance is summoned. Environmental assessment while providing discharge instruction will take on increased importance for the student who has experienced the real world of some of these clients in our community.

Students in the ICU/CCU rotation may also spend a clinical day in either the outpatient hemodialysis unit or the emergency room. A required reading helps to prepare the student for these experiences, and report forms are designed to focus on objectives specific to the role of the nurse in these areas. Although more traditionally hospital-based, the emphasis for the student's rotation to these two units is on secondary and tertiary levels of prevention through assessments and delivery of emergency or intensive care to outpatients. Since the majority of clients return home following treatment, the teaching role of the nurse is a primary focus.

Home Care Lab   A simulated home care visit was designed as a two-session laboratory in the Nursing Skills Center. The lab begins with viewing and discussing the film *Effective Home Visiting Techniques* (University of Colorado School of Nursing, 1996). In small groups, student are given a home care referral for a patient with multiple nursing problems. Students review the patient data, plan care prior to the visit, and role-play a visit to the patient's "home." Lab instructors guide student learning, supervise skill performances and bag technique, and may even fill in as the patient's family caregiver. The lab was designed by a lab instructor who worked part-time as a community health nurse and patterned the case studies on her typical patient population. The lab was introduced late in the fourth semester but will be moved to the second semester to provide a practice segment to the theory component of Community Health Nursing.

OUTCOMES

To evaluate the learning outcomes of our community infusion project, a one page questionnaire was developed. Students rated the 37 community placements and their degree of learning about the three levels of prevention on a 4-point Likert scale. In addition, they were asked what aspects of the experiences enhanced or detracted from their clinical learning and whether they thought the community experiences should be expanded or not. Results from the class of 1996 were that a large majority of the sites were rated good or excellent, and over 90 percent of the students said the community experiences helped them to understand the three levels of prevention. Write-in responses indicated that the experiences enhanced their clinical learning by introducing them to different kinds of nursing, by emphasizing the teaching role and communication skills of the nurse, and by increasing their understanding of economic diversity. A few students said the experiences detracted from their clinical learning by taking valuable time from practicing skills. Others said that the visits interrupted the continuity of the hospital portion of the rotation. Some felt that observational experiences should be limited to the freshman level. A majority of the students recommended expanding the experiences.

We are pleased with student response to the community-based experiences. Since change is often not well received, it has been pleasant to receive positive student feedback on a faculty decision believed necessary to advance learning. Another faculty objective was to widen the students' options for employment opportunities. They are acutely aware of the changing job market and change in location for delivery of health care services that was reflected in the surveys. The college conducts graduate and employer surveys every three to five years; therefore, it will be several years before we will have outcome assessments based on graduate competencies. By graduation in May 1996, one new graduate had secured employment in a community site visited during a clinical rotation, so for that one person these curricular changes made a significant difference.

FUTURE PLANS

Funding for a part-time community coordinator was obtained from the college foundation, and the original adjunct faculty member who initiated the pilot project was selected for the position. A job description for the community coordinator has been developed using guidelines established in the grant proposal (see Figure 11–2).

Organization of the community experiences, consolidation and distribution of information and revision of existing objectives and forms will be an ongoing process. A new Community Database using Gordon's 11 patterns has been designed as an all-purpose report form to simplify paperwork for students and provide continuity of the structural framework (see Figure 11–3). The major clinical additions for the 1996–1997 year are several community experiences in the second semester of the freshman year to enhance class content on adherence, and chronic and infectious diseases. Students will visit wound care and diabetic outpatient clinics focusing on tertiary prevention and on motivational communication techniques. They will also participate in tuberculosis and sexually transmitted disease clinics and make home visits to patients with AIDS,

Figure 11–2
Job Description for Community Coordinator

1. Develop a framework/model of community nursing.
2. Develop evaluation tools to measure project and student learning.
3. Call agencies to inquire about placements, experiences available, and hours.
4. Be specific about objectives of the experience and activities of students.
5. Clarify school's role in student supervision. Is on-site required by agency, school?
6. Develop all-purpose contract to be used for all agencies, ideally one not needing frequent renegotiating and send to all newly negotiated placements.
7. Compile list of agencies to be used, contact person, address, phone, appropriate dress, and assignments prior to and after the experience.
8. Organize all placements on a grid by clinical rotation so you can see at a glance which agency is being used at any given time during the semester.
9. Send letters to all placements to be used at the beginning of each semester to remind agencies that clinical instructors will be calling with specific dates and names of students.
10. Provide educational in-service to faculty to emphasize key points of community education.
11. Give all instructors the list of agencies for the particular clinical rotation. Encourage them to call agencies and send names of students for specific dates.
12. Advise instructors to inform students regarding visit schedules, location, times, contact person, dress, preassignments or readings and reports to be submitted.
13. Visit participating agencies when available, especially large community efforts such as elder or school fairs, to support instructors and students.
14. Send letters to all agencies at the end of the semester to thank them for participating.
15. Confer with instructors about feedback from students.
16. Contact agencies to assess how they perceive the placements.
17. Conduct formal evaluation surveys of students and reassess placements.
18. Write final report for publication.

Figure 11–3
Community Visit Report

Student Name ——————————————— Date ———————

Community Experience ——————————————————————

    I. Health perception/health management pattern.
      a. Describe general health of individual or groups.
      b. What does individual or group do to maintain health?
      c. How safe is the environment?

    II. Nutritional/metabolic pattern.
      a. Describe general nourishment of individual/group.
      b. Describe diet of individual/group.
      c. Describe family influence.

    III. Elimination pattern.
      a. Describe bowel/bladder habits of individual/group.
      b. Describe environmental disposal of waste.

    IV. Activity/exercise pattern.
      a. Describe level of energy and activity of individual/group.
      b. Describe recreational activities.

    V. Sleep/rest pattern.
      a. Is individual or group rested and ready for daily activity?
      b. Describe sleeping space.

    VI. Cognitive/perceptual pattern.
      a. Are individual/group's vision and hearing adequate?
      b. Do concentration and orientation seem appropriate?
      c. Are there language deficits?

    VII. Self-perception/self-concept pattern.
      a. How does individual, group, neighborhood feel about itself?

    VIII. Role-relationship pattern.
      a. Does individual(s) live alone?
      b. Is group interaction harmonious or is neighborhood comfortable?
      c. Describe family/group structure.
      d. What are the problems and how are they handled?
      e. Describe interaction between health care provider and individual or group.

    IX. Sexuality-reproductive pattern.
      a. Does individual or group behavior seem age-appropriate?
      b. Describe age-specific concerns of individual or group.

    X. Coping-stress-tolerance.
      a. Describe any recent changes and reaction.
      b. Describe methods used to decrease stress.

    XI. Value-belief pattern.
      a. Does individual/group appear satisfied with life?
      b. Is religion important?

with an emphasis on the teaching role of the community nurse. The local Parish Nursing Program will include students with the volunteer nurses who conduct basic health education programs in several parochial schools in the community.

The new curriculum commenced in the Fall of 1996 at the senior level. Changes in clinical rotations include lengthening the Medical-Surgical experience to 7½ weeks. This is paired with a combined Maternal-Child rotation of the same length. The reduction of 2½ weeks from the former Obstetric and Pediatric rotations is in response to the decreasing need for acute care nursing in these specialties. The Phase II community-based focus is being retained, with the reduction occurring in the hospital segments. The remaining clinicals—Psychiatric/Substance Abuse, ICU/CCU, and Nursing Home/Management—will continue as 5-week rotations.

Home visits with a long-term home-care nurse have been added to the Nursing Home/Management rotation. In collaboration with the County Office for Aging, several flu clinics are scheduled to occur on clinical days so that students will be able to participate in administering injections. A day at the Board of Occupational Educational Services Center (BOESC) with a school nurse who works with students who are mentally retarded and emotionally dysfunctional has been added to the Psychiatric/Substance Abuse rotation. This will reinforce student learning about physical and behavioral management of children who are too impaired to be mainstreamed into regular schools.

Beginning in Fall 1996, we will require students to maintain portfolios throughout their college years. These will include data they have retained from community visits. Items from the portfolio can be used on resumes or a summary can be taken to employment interviews to demonstrate the community-based opportunities experienced during the nursing program. This should enhance the graduate's ability to demonstrate practical experience outside the institutional setting. Motivation of the faculty and education for teaching nursing outside acute care will be a focus of departmental faculty development. The coordinator will also be responsible for updating faculty on community activities and large events such as the health fairs.

An education segment to be included in the first faculty meeting of the academic year will emphasize the essential community components of the three levels of prevention, a stronger emphasis on patient teaching, and a focus on the patient-centered environment of community settings.

Subsequent offerings being planned include clinical conference techniques to incorporate community concepts, the differentiated practice role of the associate degree nurse in the community, and essential information about reimbursement and regulatory issues in community-based health care.

Our goal is to infuse community-based nursing throughout all theory and clinical components of the curriculum. This approach is intended to result in outcomes that reflect our graduates' increased knowledge and exposure to current trends in health care delivery. In future surveys, we will expect to document that graduates have increased their familiarity with community settings, seek employment and secure job placements in these settings, feel prepared to work in the community, and experience success in these expanded environments. For those who select employment in acute care settings, the expectation is that our focus on community concepts will result in graduates with enhanced ability in patient teaching, discharge planning, and referral services.

REFERENCES

Concept Media. (1993). *Cultural diversity and nursing practice: Improving client response to health care*. [Videotape]. Irvine, CA: Author.

Cookfair, J. (1996). *Nursing care in the community*. St. Louis: Mosby.

Davis, R., & McKee-Johnson, M. (1988). Do associate degree programs need community health content? *Nurse Educator, 13*(3), 27–30.

Gordon, M. (1982). *Nursing diagnosis: Process and application*. New York: McGraw-Hill.

National League for Nursing. (1990). *Educational outcomes of associate degree nursing programs: Roles and competencies*. New York: Author.

National League for Nursing. (1993). *A vision for nursing education*. National League for Nursing Position Paper. New York: Author.

Rice, R. (1996). *Home health nursing practice* (2nd ed.). St. Louis: Mosby.

Shugars, D. A., O'Neil, E. H., & Bader, J. D. (1991). *Healthy America: Practitioners for 2005, an agenda for action for U.S. health professional schools*. Durham, NC: The Pew Health Professions Commission.

University of Colorado Health Sciences Center, School of Nursing. (1996). *Effective home visiting techniques* [Videotape]. Lawrence, KS: Learner Managed Designs.

Waters, V. (Ed.). (1991). *Teaching gerontology*. New York: National League for Nursing Press.

12

Transforming the Total Curriculum to Educate the Millennium Nurse

Alma L. Mueller
Joan E. Henshaw

The Front Range Community College (FRCC) nursing program faculty committed in 1993 to initiate curricular change to meet the challenges of a transforming health care delivery system. At that time, clinical placements in acute care were changing. There was low census everywhere. Clinical agencies were reluctant to guarantee student placements because units were in the midst of chaos or closure. Managed care was changing the way and places for health care delivery. The National League for Nursing (1993) published *Vision for Nursing Education*. Everyone was talking about "community-based, community-focused" health care. The faculty was acutely aware that education as we had been presenting it for the past decade was not going to be appropriate for graduates who would be working the majority of their career lives in the 21st century. We therefore determined to design an education for what we have coined "The Millennium Nurse." This curricular change was different from changes accomplished over the previous 20 years, which had involved reconceptualization and reorganization of basically the same content. This was a more fundamental reappraisal that rooted out deeply held paradigms learned in the nursing programs we had attended, implemented in our own clinical practice, and subsequently integrated into our teaching.

Nursing faculty from two campuses of FRCC met jointly over a two-year period to design a new curriculum, which was implemented in the fall of 1995. While it took two years to design the new curriculum, there was an immediate change in the way the program was being taught. Students noticed a difference within six months of the faculty first discussing the changes needed.

> **Critical Incident:** A student who was graduating in December 1993 came into my office one day and said, with excitement, "You have really changed the way you're teaching!" I asked her what she meant. She said: "Up to this point all of you had been talking about acute care, but this semester you have talked about so many places health care is delivered. You have opened up a whole new world to me!"

CHANGE: PROCESS AND PRODUCT

Strategies

Catalysts and Questions Affecting Change   To have curricular change occur, faculty must decide change is necessary and discuss critical questions to establish the direction change will take. Good questions are, What are your community's health problems? Where is nursing practiced today and where will it be practiced in 5 to 10 years?

During our discussion of these questions, FRCC faculty became intensely aware that we unconsciously held a perspective of the patient being only in acute care. We therefore developed a model to reframe our thinking (see Figure 12–1).

Once we consciously began reframing our teaching to include this full spectrum of health care delivery, our conceptualization of nursing content expanded, and new clinical sites began cropping up everywhere, from the independent senior citizens club, to organ donation programs, to radiology labs, to teen pregnancy programs, to a camp in the mountains for seniors. The list has grown exponentially because our minds reframed the education we deliver.

While the buzzwords are "community based and focused," we looked more to the broad spectrum of health care as seen in Figure 12–1. The curriculum is based in community because the starting point is, "What are our community's health problems?" and "Where in our community is health care provided?"

> **Pause for Reflection:** If we narrowly conceptualize "community" as home health and only add home health to our curriculum without looking to all the

Figure 12–1
FRCC Health Care Delivery Spectrum

HEALTH CARE DELIVERY

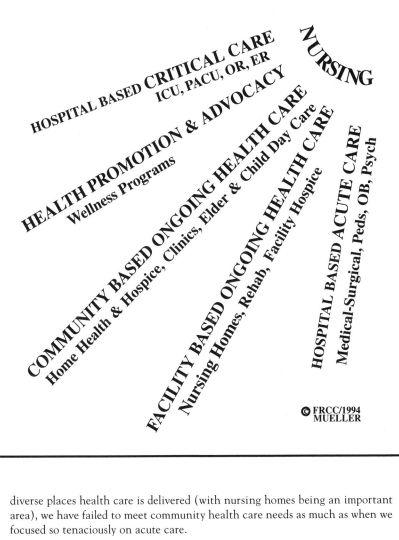

© FRCC/1994
MUELLER

diverse places health care is delivered (with nursing homes being an important area), we have failed to meet community health care needs as much as when we focused so tenaciously on acute care.

Faculty must discuss further questions: What are the most important outcomes of your nursing educational program today and what is needed for future practice? How can these outcomes be best taught in clinical and community settings and in the college classroom and lab? Wherever faculty discussions lead, the learning package of a timely curriculum must deliver certain elements universal to health care in the United States today. These elements include gerontological nursing, culturally competent care, economics and health care, and technology and informatics.

Moving from the community in general to the nursing community, another question arises: What must nursing education at every level do to promote upward educational mobility for nurses? Articulation and differentiated practice must be addressed philosophically and practically. With 32 percent of 1995 graduates from practical nursing programs and 41 percent from associate degree programs (Educational Testing Service, 1995), most new graduates are potentially available for articulation. Movement for LPNs to ADN or ADN/Diploma to BSN should include a maximum of two full-time semesters of nursing course work, potentially include a 1- to 2-credit transition course, and be available without testing applicants to prove competence.

Entropy and the Change Process   In the midst of curricular change, it is helpful to know the faculty and program director may feel uncertain, upset, helpless, or angry. Answers of *how* to change are perceived to be elusive. This is part of entropy and the change process (see Figure 12–2). Prior to change, relative harmony exists, but once the decision to change is determined and change itself is on the table, chaos prevails. With time, however, a higher order harmony is achieved. Unless one understands that chaos is part of change, one cannot believe resolution and higher order functioning will most certainly come at an undetermined and unplanned moment. When feeling the chaos, look to the entropy model in Figure 12–2; use its truth to calm anxieties. Remind the entire group of this model. Draw it on the board. It makes for a good, calming chuckle.

Changes Made by Front Range Community College

Further critical questions for the faculty are, What should be added to the curriculum? What should be deleted/cut back from the curriculum?

Decision Making   It is extremely easy to decide what to add to the curriculum, but it is very difficult to decide what to delete—and it is obvious that there must be deletions somewhere. This process is very painful

Figure 12–2
Entropy and the Change Process

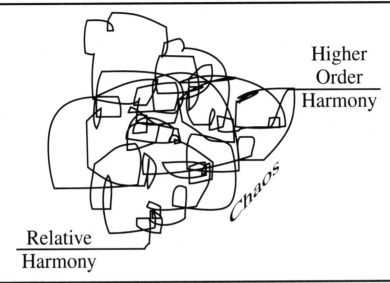

Higher
Order
Harmony

Chaos

Relative
Harmony

for those faculty who teach in areas that will be deleted or significantly shortened. However, the earlier questions will help them see that change is necessary and that they can learn how to teach new areas in the curriculum.

It is also critical that faculty do not unwittingly cut back on areas that are major health problems in their community. Always return to the original questions and discussion to analyze the appropriateness of areas to delete or cut back.

> **Critical Incidents:** At one curricular change workshop, a faculty member said she could cut back on the amount of time spent on drug abuse. Yet how could content on drug abuse be decreased when it remains a major community health problem? At another school, faculty talked about cutting back on gerontological nursing. Yet our older population is growing at a fast rate and requires more health care than other age groups. These are not reasonable areas to downsize.

Once faculty have fully discussed what to add and delete, the decision then must be made whether to create an entirely new curriculum or to significantly alter what is already in place. FRCC faculty chose the latter. We kept most courses as they were (credit hours, content guides) while making major changes in how we approached learning in those courses (whether lab, clinical placement, clinical teaching, or classroom content), deleted parts of other courses, and created several new courses.

> *Pause for Reflection:* If only a few courses in the curriculum are changed without an altered mind-set in all the faculty who teach the curriculum, a program will not have a transformed curriculum. Altering the mind-set includes:
>
> - Thinking about what constitutes the community's health problems.
> - Moving away from an unconscious and unyielding orientation to acute care while moving toward the full spectrum of health care delivery.
> - Teaching to program outcomes in every course rather than focusing first and foremost on course content.
> - Reframing how we approach teaching—or rather "learning."

Areas Deleted from the Curriculum   Based on faculty discussion of the key questions, we chose to delete some of the time spent in our specialty areas. We decreased the total credit hours in maternal and child nursing by 27 percent and mental health nursing by 14 percent. The decrease was in clinical/laboratory time rather than classroom time. We did not eliminate clinical learning in these areas, we decreased it.

Areas Added to the Curriculum: New First-Year Courses

1. A new 1-credit laboratory course was designed to present beginning concepts of assessment, communication, and teaching.
2. An existing first-year adult nursing clinical course was restructured with additional credit to enhance gerontological nursing. The new content in this course includes (1) a seminar focusing on our aging population; (2) a community-based practicum centered on communication and teaching involving a series of visits to a well elder living independently, and (3) a nursing home practicum.

New Second-Year Nursing Courses

1. A 2-credit gerontological nursing course was developed. The course has three components:
   - A seminar focuses on gerontological assessment including normal versus abnormal changes for the older adult and differences

in the ways older adults present with illness; specific disease processes such as delirium, dementia, and Alzheimer's; appropriate use of therapies such as validation, reminiscence, reality orientation, and remotivation; nursing care specific to the home setting; and methods of reimbursement and cost containment.

- A nursing home clinical provides students the opportunity to refine their gerontological assessment skills, practice rehabilitation and restorative nursing care, implement therapeutic modalities, and apply principles of delegation.

- A home health clinical provides a one-day observational experience with a home health nurse. Students identify preparation required for home health visits, discuss RN responsibilities in home care, and explore adaptation of nursing procedures to the home setting.

2. A second 2-credit course was designed to allow students to focus on a specific area of health care delivery. Students are equally divided among the five rays in our health care delivery spectrum (see Figure 12–1) for their 5-day clinical experience.

Before the clinical experience begins, students prepare written papers on issues and on cognitive, affective, and psychomotor skills related to the selected clinical setting. Within the setting, students implement nursing care, and identify and address a potential area of conflict exploring negotiation and conflict resolution. In a formal 30-minute classroom presentation, students teach peers and faculty about their area of health care delivery. This course provides a foundation to better coordinate care across the health delivery spectrum, because students learn how clients access and move around the system. It also teaches students how to deliberately and systematically seek knowledge in new areas of nursing care delivery.

Exposing Students to the Full Spectrum of Health Care Delivery It is critical to provide a variety of clinical sites within the total curriculum. However, the setting for a given course is not necessarily critical because we are teaching the program outcomes within the broad spectrum of delivery sites; objectives driven by settings are a secondary focus. Consequently, settings for given courses can change as communities change.

We have designed our curriculum with built-in flexibility. As nursing care evolves and shifts to different settings in our communities, we can redirect didactic and clinical content in existing courses to these new settings while maintaining our focus on the outcomes expected. This has already occurred because the rehabilitation settings that were initially available to us underwent multiple mergers and changed in focus. We have easily moved from one type of setting to another since our focus is on student outcomes delivered in various settings.

Changing Faculty Roles

What feelings do these curricular changes evoke in faculty? In attempting to adjust to this transformed curriculum, faculty may sometimes feel completely overwhelmed. Allowing faculty to openly discuss feelings pulls them together and moves them forward. In the clinical arena, moving from teaching in acute care to other areas requires learning new content—new expertise—related to what clients are like and how care is delivered. It also demands new clinical teaching styles because teaching in acute care is largely reactive; faculty react to fast-paced changes in clients, their family dynamics, and procedures ordered. Teaching in other areas is more directional and involves working with our nurse colleagues in different ways from those used in acute care.

In the past, "units" with numerous patients, where we could have full student groups supervised by one faculty on site, was our major mode of teaching. Now, students will be in numerous sites, precepted by nurses at those sites and coordinated by a faculty from the college. This requires us to rethink how we determine a student to be competent and successfully achieving the program outcomes and clinical objectives. These changes require serious paradigm shifts for faculty. In the classroom, we have been looking at changing teaching styles for a number of years. In moving from the lecture mode to interactive classroom activities, faculty can no longer ask how to improve teaching, but rather how to cause learning.

When *anyplace* in the community is utilized for student learning, faculty must be heavily involved in acquiring clinical learning sites. With the use of dialysis centers, home care, mall clinics, Head Start, homeless shelters, and other numerous possibilities, program director and faculty roles for designing and acquiring placements are merging. Program directors must determine ways to make this acquisition of clinicals part of the teaching load and not merely add this task on top of current faculty responsibilities.

Front Range Community College Nursing Education Model

The FRCC nursing faculty spent time during the change process discussions to develop a nursing education model that reflected our philosophy (see Figure 12–3). The three main beliefs represented in the model are an affirmation of student and nurse diversity, a belief in nursing educational articulation, and delivery of nursing care across the health care spectrum.

Front Range Community College Graduate Outcomes and Curricular Framework

The FRCC faculty spent two days establishing outcomes we wanted to instill in our graduates for the 21st century. We determined our outcomes with the help of a consultant, and then used the Nominal Group Technique to resolve what the outcomes meant to us. This technique emphasizes equality of ideas, ensures no ideas are lost, and diminishes the impact of a dominant person (Delbeq, VandeVen, & Gustasson, 1975, quoted by Higgins, 1994, pp. 150–153).

Figure 12–3
FRCC Nursing Education Model

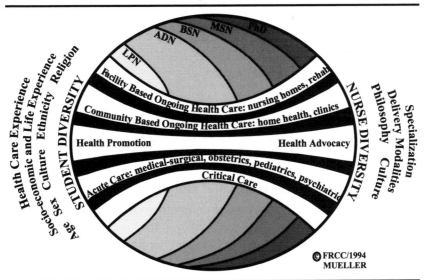

Critical Incident: By collaboratively interpreting outcomes, faculty were able to truly embed those outcomes in the curriculum. Student assignments across the curriculum changed in various creative ways to direct the students to look at how they were implementing the outcomes. An example is the strategy of second-year students journaling to the outcomes during clinical rotations. This encouraged students to look at competencies they were acquiring rather than focusing on discrete tasks, events, or knowledge.

The FRCC program outcomes are caring, clinically competent, communicator/collaborator, teacher/learner, critical thinker, and professional. Beyond the more traditional definitions of these outcomes, faculty specifically chose to include the following as major components of those outcomes: Caring includes culturally sensitive care; clinically competent includes age-appropriate (old as well as young) and culturally competent care; communicator/collaborator includes negotiation skills and communication with colleagues and community; teacher/learner includes lifelong learning; critical thinker includes change as constant; and professional includes the realities of economics and health care.

Another area in our curriculum needing reframing was our approach to the goal of nursing care. At a conference presented by the Medical College of Pennsylvania and Hahnemann University, Elaine Tagliareni from the Community College of Philadelphia discussed the power of utilizing *client optimal functioning* (Tagliareni, 1995). This presentation was exciting for our faculty because, again, it reframed our thinking. Once we put optimal functioning at the center of our curricular framework, *nursing* flowed. It drove us away from the medical model toward a nursing model that centered not on illness, but on the impact illness and prevention of illness had for that patient and family. When this became the core of our framework, students and faculty alike moved toward the client as the center of care, and brought creative and holistic nursing to help clients achieve their own life goals. Students began to truly envision the client beyond the dressing change as an individual able to make choices, involved in health care, fulfilling dreams, and having wisdom.

The FRCC nursing curriculum framework (see Figure 12–4) places the client's outcome of optimal functioning at the core, supported by student outcomes learned in the program, and implemented everywhere in the health care spectrum. The model resembles a flower, unfolding as students learn outcomes throughout the program.

Figure 12–4
FRCC Nursing Program Framework

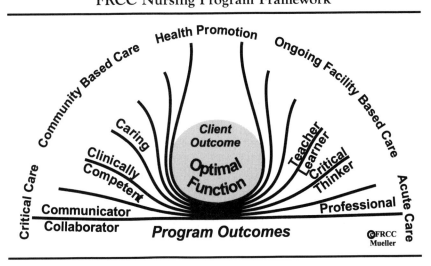

NUTS AND BOLTS

The Millennium Nurse must possess higher level cognitive and affective skills to succeed in the community-focused system that lies ahead. Certain learning strategies threaded throughout a curriculum facilitate the skills. The FRCC nursing faculty have implemented their threads in a deliberate manner that continues to unfold as this content is taught. In this section, we will share some of our approaches with you.

Mandatory Study/Work Groups

All nursing students are required to become part of a study/work group. These groups were initially conceptualized to function in two ways: to promote critical thinking and to acquire collaborative skills.

Study/work groups are formed at a mandatory, noncredit, daylong student success workshop before nursing classes begin. This workshop includes activities designed to practice techniques of relaxation and imagery, to incorporate critical thinking skills, and to foster positive relationships with peers. Students get to know one another using icebreaking techniques. By midday, they self-select into study/work groups with eight members.

This study/work group is then assigned as the first laboratory/clinical rotation group. After the first rotation, students are assigned to clinicals randomly. Although students initially dislike being away from their friends in these new rotations, they soon interact with other peers and find they grow with the new support.

Most study/work groups continue unchanged during the two years, successfully working out intragroup issues and problems. However, much like work groups in the real world, a few of the study/work groups disintegrate and these students merge with other groups.

After working with study/work groups for more than two years, we found them to be powerful. In addition to accomplishing the first two goals, other positive by-products emerged. These included easy formation of task groups, quicker and better group problem-solving, crossover of collaborative skills to new groups, built-in support for "loners," and better resolution of student/faculty issues.

Communication with Colleagues and Community

Nursing programs have traditionally focused on client and family communication techniques. With programs becoming community-focused, program requirements and student objectives related to communication must broaden. Student-initiated communication in the community must explore joint needs and be goal directed—especially when faculty are not available on site.

> **Critical Incident:** A student was collecting data from the community on the pro-choice/abortion issue. In meeting with staff of a Planned Parenthood office, the student interrogated more than interviewed. Because the questions were controversial and the staff did not know exactly what the student wanted, the police were called and so were we. (We won't discuss the time former Governor Lamm called us.) We hope that broadening objectives to include communication techniques with the community will prevent recurrence of similar situations!

Another facet of communication, identified by nurse administrators, includes a need for new graduates to better handle conflict situations with a variety of health care staff.

Collaboration and Negotiation Skills

To collaborate effectively, people must have adequate self-esteem. We use several methods to enhance self-esteem. At several intervals in the curriculum, students are taught to utilize positive affirmations to increase success. Negative thoughts are reworded to be positive statements.

> *Example:* Instead of "I am trying to pass the test," the student is encouraged to think, "I have the necessary information and tools to answer the questions correctly."

We also enhance self-esteem by facilitating students with major life issues to briefly state the problem(s) and move quickly to their own solutions. We found that listening to students' ongoing "Ain't It Awful" speeches and providing solutions was counterproductive for adult learners and faculty. We now help students seek their own solutions versus handing them solutions. Students who have learned new ways to problem-solve have subsequently become more successful in working with colleagues.

Additionally, we encourage students to learn how to promote self-esteem in others. We teach students to evaluate each other in the lab. Students ask their peers first to self-evaluate, and then the student evaluators provide a feedback "sandwich" of positives surrounding any negatives. There is a role change for faculty from evaluator to teacher of evaluation that isn't easy and takes practice. For too long we have been quick to judge. Making the evaluator role a shared responsibility empowers nurses to work as colleagues.

In promoting the role of colleague, beginning students are encouraged to ask questions of peers, instructors, and staff using a nondefensive approach:

> *Example:* From a student to the nurse: "Did you plan to get Mr. Jones up later?" Instead of: "Why isn't Mr. Jones up in his chair?"

At the beginning of the second year, faculty and students participate in a highly interactive off-campus workshop. For two days, students learn skills of assertiveness, negotiation, and group decision making in experiential situations. Brief lectures, role-playing, skits, and problem-solving are used to learn how to send "I" messages, attack the problem instead of the people, and handle difficult situations.

Broad-Based Assessment

The FRCC nursing faculty have been continually committed to holistic caring. As health broadens its spectrum of delivery, comprehensive client assessments are a necessity. Instead of focusing narrowly on immediate client problems or on physical assessment, students must examine the larger picture to achieve realistic optimal functioning for the client (e.g., the client will be able to attend Bingo games versus only focusing on solving the problem of changing a sterile dressing over a nasty wound).

Throughout the nursing program, students utilize a faculty-generated data collection tool to perform broad-based assessment. This comprehensive assessment guide is modified from Maslow's basic human needs and also includes aspects of a mental status exam, functional assessment, environment, knowledge deficits, culture, and spirituality. Client information includes prior and current lifestyle patterns.

Critical Thinking

Along with other programs across the country, we are infusing critical thinking into the curriculum. As illustrated in the following examples, we are actively seeking and implementing innovative techniques:

- Based on a technique described by Marianne Malagne (personal communication) from the North Harris Montgomery Community College district in Houston, we have our students learn how to don sterile gloves using critical thinking skills. Without seeing a live demonstration or video, the students are given simple guidelines (e.g., "Keep the outside of these gloves sterile while putting them on"). After a student group has decided how to don the gloves, the instructor facilitates the group in evaluating their technique. Some student groups successfully accomplish the task through shared discussion, whereas others need instructor assistance to enhance their skills of observation and problem-solving. Some students tend to convince themselves they are right and are surprised when the practiced eye of the instructor detects a problem. These students need assistance to look at more than one solution and to view making errors as an opportunity to learn, not as a failure.

- Increased delegation of nursing skills means nurses must assess the performance of other caregivers. For selected fundamentals and med-surg procedures, FRCC students are asked to evaluate each others' performance with instructor supervision. Students "see one, do one, and evaluate one." Students analyze performance based on scientific principles while utilizing positive communication techniques to give feedback. This requires higher level thinking.

- Collaborative testing is used in a number of courses throughout the curriculum. After students have turned in individual answer sheets, the study/work group then takes the exam collaboratively. Items engendering disagreement among the group are discussed using critical thinking skills. We have found students clarify their own thinking and learn from each other when they provide their peers with rationale for their choice of answer.

- To increase the students' critical thinking skills in classroom, lab, and clinical, faculty ask, "What led to your conclusion? What could you have done differently to accomplish the same goal or a different outcome? What other information or ideas did you consider and discard in coming to this conclusion?" Answering these questions helps students validate their thinking process.

Teaching "Teaching" across the Curriculum

Several teaching projects are deliberately placed in every semester of the nursing program:

- In the first semester, student study/work groups present cultural beliefs and customs of the five most common cultural groups in our community. Afterward, a potluck dinner with food from each of the five cultures is shared.

- In the second semester, student groups present ethical dilemmas related to the elderly through a role-playing/skit/debate format followed by further presentation and discussion.

- In the third semester, student groups employ creative ideas to present skits in pharmacology encompassing such topics as drug side effects, client teaching in diverse settings, and drug physiology.

- In the fourth semester, each student gives a formal 30-minute presentation about his or her clinical assignment in the spectrum of health care delivery. Visual aids and audience participation are techniques used in presenting.

The purpose of infusing teaching projects in every semester goes beyond learning how to teach. Presenting group projects fosters critical thinking, creativity, clarity, and collaboration. It also fosters self confidence.

> **Critical Incident:** A relatively shy student in her final clinical experience came in excitedly one day and said she found herself saying really great things in clinical to other nurses and doctors. Her ability to be articulate really surprised her. Ideas sounded so good, she found herself turning around to see who had said them. She suddenly realized she was able to express her ideas so well because of all the skits and presentations she had done during the program. She thanked us for making her do all those teaching projects that she had so hated at the time!

FUTURE PLANS

Our primary plan is to see change as constant—to teach it and live it.

We are currently integrating nursing informatics and technology deliberately into the curriculum and planning to participate in a differentiated practice project similar to the Healing Web project in South Dakota. We intend to expand our community focus, better implement critical thinking skills, and facilitate collaboration for students and faculty. We choose to innovate, experiment, revise, and revitalize—and withhold judgment. We are never done. We are consciously learning to gracefully accept change and to survive in a climate of chaos and complexity.

May our vision be clear, our entropy manageable, our time infinite, and our universe expanding.

REFERENCES

Delbeq, A. L., VandeVen, A. H., & Gustasson, D. H. (1975). *Group techniques for program planning.* Glenview, IL: Scott Foresman, quoted by Higgins, J. M. (1994). *101 creative problem solving techniques.* New York: New Management.

Educational Testing Service. (1995). *Quarterly reports.* Princeton, NJ: Author.

National League for Nursing. (1993, June). *Vision for nursing education.* New York: Author.

Tagliareni, E. (1995). Speech presented at Dimensions in Academic Leadership: An Institute for ADN Administrators. Orlando, FL: Medical College of Pennsylvania.

13

Here Comes the Neighborhood

The Northeastern University Curriculum Model of Community-Based Education

Barbara Kelley
Mary Anne Gauthier
Peggy S. Matteson
Margaret Ann Mahoney

Curriculum changes in nursing education must keep pace with the rapid changes in the health care delivery system in the United States. Today's nursing students will be responsible for providing and managing patient care in an evolving health care delivery system. As nursing educators, we must empower nursing students to understand the forces driving these changes, to appreciate the implications that changes in the health care delivery system will have on patient care, and to embrace and manage change.

Health care delivery changes are being driven by a powerful force called finances, more particularly by big businesses that no longer want to pay exorbitant health care premiums and Wall Street investors who want cost-efficient health care companies. This is a very different set of forces from the altruistic and paternalistic view of health care that has existed over the past century. Hospitals, the traditional place for patients to receive care, no longer play the pivotal role they once did in the health care delivery system. The health care paradigm is shifting, hospitals are downsizing and mergers are occurring.

With an ever-increasing amount of health care being provided outside the acute care institution, how can we teach students what they need to know to become capable nurses? Nurse educators can no longer rely on the traditional and predominantly hospital-based teaching model. Future nurses must be educated within the larger, more encompassing community-based perspective of nursing and health care. Nursing education can no longer be setting specific. The focus of nurse educators must be that nursing occurs wherever the nurse and the patient are located. This concept is the catalyst in the transformation of nursing education to a community-based approach.

COMMUNITY-BASED CURRICULUM CHANGE

One example of curriculum change to a primary care, community-based focus has occurred within the Northeastern University's College of Nursing in Boston, Massachusetts. The College of Nursing faculty, supported in part by a Kellogg Foundation grant, worked over a five-year span to significantly change the nursing curriculum. The current curriculum is designed to provide 50 percent of the students' clinical experiences in a community setting.

CHALLENGES

Change does not come easily. The shift from traditional practices and proven educational methods carries with it challenges and risks. One challenge is to find meaningful clinical experiences that provide the students with opportunities to learn the knowledge, skills, and attitudes necessary to the practice of nursing. Another challenge is to excite the faculty to develop and embrace new modes of teaching. With rapid patient turnover, there is the risk that clinical experiences in any arena will not meet the expectations of faculty and/or students. The greater risk, however, lies in not creatively preparing students to understand the changing health care system, in not preparing students to be effective nurses in the 21st century.

SYSTEM CHANGES

The shift from hospital-based to community-based nursing education is grounded in the realities of the changing health care delivery system, but it does not alter the foundational values of nursing: caring, communication, critical thinking, clinical judgment, and therapeutic interventions.

The focus remains on the patient and provision of nursing care regardless of the practice site. The move to primary care/managed care is, in fact, a more powerful model of care for nursing interventions. Nurses can engage patients as partners in their care. Teaching health education and disease prevention as well as supporting patients in self-care is a primary role of nurses. Managed care systems, in the business of managing costs, look to prevention as the key to avoiding costly illness and prolonged social interventions.

The paradigm shift in nursing education is one of changing systems. Nursing faculty, along with the majority of practicing nurses, have been part of an institutional, bureaucratic system where patients delivered themselves or were delivered to the hospital and turned over to providers for care. Nurses have been taught to use their critical thinking, clinical judgment, and decision-making skills within a closed, self-contained system. When a patient needed a referral, it was a phone call away. When new medication was needed, the pharmacy delivered it. When X-rays or other interventions were ordered, the patient was transported to the appropriate department and returned to his or her assigned room within a short time frame. Providing nursing care to a patient in a hospital setting depended on the nurse thoroughly understanding how the system worked as well as being able to interact with the patient and the family. Nursing expertise became synonymous with both system and patient.

Hospital or institutional-based care further defined the patient's need for nursing care in an artificial way. Care was episodic and removed from the totality of the patient's family, community, and cultural orientation. Patients went to the hospital because of an illness, surgery, or trauma. The nursing care learned by students revolved around treating the patient's condition, educating and supporting the patient in self-care, and preparing the patient for discharge.

Moving nursing education out into the community requires nursing students to problem-solve in a different kind of system. Caring for a patient in the community requires knowledge of the community support system. Where is the pharmacy that supplies the patient's medication? Is it a short walk away? What are the operating hours? How far does a patient have to travel for an X-ray or ultrasound? Does it require a bus or cab ride and can the patient afford it? Who shops or provides transportation for the patient when he or she cannot or will not? Is there any family support? Are there any helpful neighbors? If the patient comes from a different cultural background, is there an identified social group to turn to for help?

FACULTY VALUES

It was this system change approach that presented the biggest challenge to the faculty and to curriculum change at Northeastern University. How could we ensure that nursing students would become socialized into the profession of nursing and acquire the needed technical skills in a system that was the domain of the community health nursing specialist? How could faculty members who were not community health specialists teach students in a community setting? How can anyone be a nurse without a defining "med-surg" experience? What kind of learning would take place in the community if the students were out of sight and/or control of the nursing faculty (Matteson, 1995)?

After much discussion, the decision was made to provide 50 percent of the students' clinical experiences in the community setting. The other 50 percent of clinical experiences were designed to occur in the more traditional institutional settings such as acute care hospitals, long-term care, and rehabilitative settings. The move to a community-based model of nursing education does not negate the need for hospital-based clinical experiences. In fact, because patients are prepared in their community for a hospital experience and are returned "quicker and sicker" back to their community, the students benefit from understanding the value and intricacies of both systems of care. The faculty also decided that curriculum change would embrace the total curriculum and involve every student. The community-based experiences could not be limited to a selected group of students as a pilot project. If the faculty truly believed in the paradigm shift in health care delivery, it was essential that each student be prepared to practice in the multiple settings where patients would be found.

COMMUNITY PARTNERSHIPS

For community-based education to be successful, it is necessary for the faculty to identify what is meant by community or neighborhood. Does the neighborhood have geographic boundaries? Is the neighborhood divided by highways or isolated by water? Does the community have demographic characteristics (e.g., an ethnic or cultural group) that cross boundaries? Geographic maps, political district designations, bus route maps, zip codes and area codes are all useful tools in defining a community base (Matteson, 1995, pp. 54–81).

In addition to identifying a community area, it is essential to identify community partners in the educational process. This requires that the nursing faculty agree on the concept of partnership in nursing education. Can individuals other than nurse educators be involved in nursing education? Can nursing students learn about health, illness, and systems of care from other health professionals, family members, or patients? If so, then community partners need to be identified. At Northeastern University, community partners include nurses, physicians, community outreach workers, educators, project coordinators, and community members. Of necessity, the next question becomes, what is the role of nursing faculty and what role will the community partners play?

Defining Partnership

Northeastern University's community-based program is a negotiated partnership that is mutually beneficial to the College of Nursing and the communities. The participating neighborhood health centers in Boston were excited about the prospect of educating nursing, medical, and other health professions students. It was important, however, for the academicians to understand that the communities were invested in providing educational opportunities for these students in a way that was helpful to the communities. This was not to be a project where academia would come in and say to the communities, "This is what we can do for you." It was to be a project with mutually agreed on educational goals and objectives. The communities were to identify how the students could be of benefit to them as the students spent time learning with community members.

Community Values

A partnership requires shared control over clinical learning experiences. Both the university's administration and faculty had to trust that community health care providers, board members, and community activists could identify health issues within their own communities. The community people had to trust that the university faculty would build a curriculum allowing the students to meet the communities' needs and be of service in their learning experiences.

Community members were also concerned with many students coming and going in the community. To minimize intrusions into well-established, often small, neighborhood health facilities, it was agreed that student participation would comprise consistency and longevity. Nursing students are assigned to a community in their first clinical experience. In each of the subsequent clinical experiences over the next four years, the students return to "their community" for an assigned clinical experience or to do clinical projects. This curriculum design has worked very well. The community members and the students have a shared sense of ownership in the educational and caregiving process. People in the community look forward to and welcome the nursing students as they return for clinical experiences, and the students become comfortable and knowledgeable about the community and its members. By revisiting some of the same community sites, such as the schools, shelters, or homes, the students are able to build on earlier knowledge and skills and see a progression in their ability to make more complete assessments and provide more skilled care (Matteson, 1995).

NORTHEASTERN UNIVERSITY CURRICULUM

The College of Nursing at Northeastern University is a five-year cooperative program built on an academic quarter system. Students are accepted directly into the College of Nursing and nursing courses are offered during the five years of matriculation (see Tables 13–1 and 13–1A). Introductory nursing and clinical skills courses are offered in the first year of the program. These beginning nursing courses are designed to help the students conceptualize and practice nursing care regardless of the patient setting. Nurses from a variety of community and institutional settings are invited to speak to the students in the introductory and foundational courses. The students have a health assessment course with a skills lab that uses community-based case studies as a teaching methodology. One example of this methodology is in teaching students how to bathe a patient. Students are put in groups of three, in which they role-play patient, family member, and nurse. The "nurse" must teach the "family member" how to bathe the "patient." This case-based teaching actively engages the students in critical thinking, communication, teaching, and physical assessment while learning multiple nursing roles and skills.

Clinical Experiences

Clinical experiences in the community can occur in a variety of settings as long as they meet the course objectives. In the second year, students

Table 13–1
Northeastern University College of Nursing Baccalaureate
Program in Nursing Course Descriptions 1996–1997

NUR 1102   Introduction to Human Nutrition   4QH
Explores the fundamental role of nutrition in promoting health. Studies the physiological functions of nutrients, their food sources, and recommended intakes for different groups. Uses principles from the humanities and sciences in developing nutrition concepts. Introduces the use of diet assessment tools to assist individuals in meeting nutrient and energy needs. Encourages students to examine their own food choices and how those choices translate into meeting recommended nutrient and energy needs. Discusses the origins of food habits and the relevance of nutrition counseling and education in nursing practice.

NUR 1106   Introduction to Professional Nursing   2QH
Focuses on socializing students to the discipline of nursing with an introduction to theory-based practice and the philosophy of caring. Explores the dimensions of the professional role within the context of the student's developing self-awareness of personal and professional goals.

NUR 1107   Nursing Process and Skills   3QH
Emphasizes the centrality of critical thinking to clinical reasoning. Introduces the nursing process as a problem-solving tool and its application in assessing strategies of communication, gathering data, interpreting evidence, analyzing viewpoints, and forming judgments. Provides scientific principles as the framework for using basic nursing skills in the practice of selected nursing interventions. Includes practicing skills in a clinical laboratory. *Prereq. or concurrent NUR 1106*

NUR 1108   Nursing Health Assessment   3QH
Emphasizes dimensions of collecting data relevant to health status. Provides an opportunity for learning to use tools and skills of health assessment. Discusses ethnic, cultural, spiritual, social, psychological, development, gender, and physical aspects of health assessment. Explores formulating nursing diagnosis and examining the relationship of the nursing care plan to overall resources of the client. Includes practicing skills in a clinical laboratory. *Prereq. or concurrent NUR 1106*

NUR 1202   Pathophysiological Concepts for Clinical Nursing   4QH
Reviews human physiology related to oxygenation, nutrition, elimination, protective mechanisms, neurological functions, endocrine functions, and skin integrity. Explores how the human body uses its adaptive powers to maintain equilibrium and how alterations affect normal processes. Examines disease processes and implications for nursing practice. *Prereq. BIO 1154 or equivalent*

NUR 1206   Promoting Healthy Childbearing and Childrearing   8QH
Emphasizes the promotion of health from conception to adolescence. Describes potential and actual health risk factors and explores risk reduction strategies within the context of the individual, family, and community. Uses the nursing process to provide

(Continued)

Table 13–1 (*Continued*)

the framework for students to assess and intervene therapeutically in promoting healthy childbearing and childrearing. Examines the concepts of human development of the individual, family and community within the context of the role of the professional nurse in promoting healthy childbearing and childrearing. Includes clinical learning experiences in a variety of settings. *Prereq. NUR 1107, 1108*

NUR 1208   Promoting Healthy Adulthood and Aging   8QH
Emphasizes the promotion of health in adults and includes common health problems of adults at critical life stages from the young adult to the frail elderly years. Analyzes potential and actual health risk factors and the discovery of risk reduction strategies by applying the nursing process to care of adults living within families and communities. Enables students to use health education and teaching methods in assessing and intervening therapeutically to meet the primary health care needs of adults. Assesses the role of the nurse in partnership with the family and community in disease prevention. Includes clinical learning experiences in a variety of settings. *Prereq. NUR 1206*

NUR 1282   Wellness   4QH
Focuses on experiential exploration of the concept of wellness. Examines behaviors and lifestyle choices that lead to a high level of physical, emotional, and spiritual well-being. Includes issues of assessment of health risk, behavior change, lifestyle analysis, the life cycle, and stress management through self analysis. *Open to any undergraduate student.*

NUR 1304   Independent Study Elective   2QH
Allows students to pursue a topic more intensely or with a special focus. Enables student to contract with a faculty member whose background, interests, and time allow direction of in-depth study. Requires that student and faculty member jointly develop course objectives.

NUR 1306   Promoting Health Restoration in Children   10QH
Focuses on the therapeutic nursing interventions used to restore health to children who are experiencing acute or chronic health problems. Analyzes complex health issues within the context of the individual, family, and community. Examines altered family patterns of coping within a developmental framework and describes support to meet the unique health needs of the family and child. Addresses the therapeutic role in partnership with the family and resources available within a collaborative and interdisciplinary environment. Discusses ethical and legal dimensions of caring for children and their families. Includes clinical learning experiences in a variety of settings. *Prereq. NUR 1208*

NUR 1307   Influences on Health and Disease   4QH
Enables the student to understand the values that underlie health seeking behavior and providing care. Uses values clarification to appreciate individual rights and responsibilities versus the common good. Examines cultural differences in light of individual and group behavior, as well as life span issues, family and group responsibilities. Builds a caring ethic and a sense of professional responsibility on the basis of self awareness and self-examination.

Table 13–1 (Continued)

NUR 1308   Promoting Health Restoration of Adults   10QH
Focuses on the therapeutic nursing interventions used to restore health to adults who are experiencing acute and/or complex health problems. Analyzes deviations from health with attention to the implications for the individual, as well as the family, in coping with health problems. Analyzes the client's health care needs and the resources to meet them, in collaboration with the client and health providers. Discusses ethical and legal dimensions of nursing care of adults. Emphasizes discharge planning and teaching. Includes clinical learning experiences in a variety of settings. *Prereq. NUR 1206, 1208*

NUR 1404   Nurse Entrepreneur   4QH
Focuses on the role of the nurse as an entrepreneur. Within the general functions of nursing, uses situations involving patient family teaching that provide the framework for introducing students to the essentials of undertaking this function as a business venture. Includes the formation of a nurse entrepreneur's venture action plan to do patient and family teaching. *Open to middler, junior, and senior students in nursing.*

NUR 1406   Promoting Healthy Communities   7QH
Focuses on developing, implementing, and evaluating therapeutic interventions for the community as the client. Uses the nursing process within the community context informed by epidemiological trends, sociocultural characteristics, political and legislative influences, organizational programs, environmental factors, and consumer inputs. Emphasizes the role of the public health nurse in multiple arenas of practice. Examines epidemiological principles and public health policies in relation to identified health problems and conditions in a specific community. Enables students to conduct a comprehensive assessment, in partnership with the community, to develop a program to meet an identified community health need. Includes clinical learning experiences in a variety of settings. *Prereq. NUR 1308*

NUR 1408   Promoting Mental Health Restoration   7QH
Focuses on developing, implementing, and evaluating psychotherapeutic interventions for clients with complex mental health problems. Analyzes alterations in psychobiological and psychosocial functioning and coping. Formulates a plan of care within the context of the client as individual, family, group, and community. Emphasizes the therapeutic use of self as students develop communication and other helping skills in interpersonal relationships with clients. Provides the opportunity to apply theories, principles, and research findings in providing mental health care for clients in various settings. Fosters collaboration with the client and interdisciplinary team. Discusses the political, legal and ethical issues related to the delivery of mental health services and the creative role of the nurse. Includes clinical learning experiences in a variety of settings. *Prereq. NUR 1308*

(Continued)

Table 13–1 (*Continued*)

NUR 1502   Introduction to Research in Nursing   4QH

Builds on students' prior exposure to select studies applied to nursing. Discusses and critiques qualitative and quantitative research and the value of each to the practice of nursing and to the health care field. Examines the importance of research in nursing to both practitioner and consumer. *Prereq. or concurrent SOC 1320 or equivalent*

NUR 1507   Comprehensive Nursing Practicum   6QH

Helps students to synthesize nursing knowledge, skills, and experience and facilitate their transition to professional nursing practice and case management of clients with complex health problems. Enables students to demonstrate leadership and collaborative skills in working with other members of the health care team. Examines professional, role and career issues in a weekly seminar. Includes clinical learning experiences in a variety of settings. *Prereq. Senior Standing*

NUR 1508   Managing and Leading in Nursing   6QH

Focuses on the knowledge and skills related to the delivery of health services within a nursing management context. Presents theories, concepts, and models, such as managed care, organization and management, authority, delegation, resource allocation, budgeting, leadership and empowerment, change, motivation, environmental safety, quality improvement, collective bargaining, and conflict resolution, to give the student an understanding of the knowledge base for the management role of the baccalaureate nurse. Provides the opportunity to apply principles and practice skills in planning and delegating nursing care using different organizational models and approaches. Discusses developing creative roles for managing and leading in nursing. Includes clinical learning experiences in a variety of settings. *Prereq. Senior Standing*

NUR 1600   International Health Care Practices   4QH

Introduces the student to the ways in which people in developing nations take care of their health. Considers the cultural context of health care practices, viewed within the framework of what people believe about themselves and the world around them; the relationship of individual and cultural belief systems; the role religious and spiritual beliefs play in protection, care, and curing; ideas about food and its relationship to health; the concepts of health education in a belief system; and the ethical issues of health care and resource allocation. *Open to any undergraduate student.*

NUR 1606   Women's Health Choices and Decisions   4QH

Explores personal health and safety concerns specific to women from menarche to mid-life. Helps to empower students to take charge of their health by examining personal experiences and developing their knowledge base and self-awareness. Investigates self-promotion of health; how to be a knowledgeable consumer; when and how to choose a provider; and care options for fertility regulation, infertility, pregnancy, childbirth, and other conditions specific to women. *Open to any undergraduate student.*

Table 13–1A
Northeastern University College of Nursing BSN Curriculum Plan*

Freshman Year 1995–1996

Fall	QH	Winter	QH	Spring	QH	Summer	QH
BIO 1152 Anatomy & Phys. I	4	BIO 1153 Anatomy & Phys. II	4	BIO 1154 Anatomy & Phys. III	4	VACATION	
ENG 1110 English I	4	ENG 1111 English II	4	PSY 1271 Social Psychology	4		
MTH 1101 Appl. of Algebra	4	PSY 1111 Psychology I	4	NUR 1102 Human Nutrition	4		
NUR 1106 Intro to Prof. Nsg.	2	NUR 1107 Nsg Proc. Skills	3	NUR 1108 Nsg. Hlth. Assessmnt.	3		
COP 1370 Intro. Career Mgmt.	1						
	15		15		15		

Sophomore Year 1996–1997

Fall	QH	Winter	QH	Spring	QH	Summer	QH
BIO 1120 Basic Microbiology	4	(Coop #1)		CHM 1106 Chemistry	5	(Coop #2)	
SOC 1100 Sociology	4			NUR 1307 Health & Disease	2		
NUR 1206 Healthy Childrearing	8			NUR 1208 Adulthood & Aging	10		
	16				17		

Middler Year 1997–1998

Fall	QH	Winter	QH	Spring	QH	Summer	QH
(Coop #3)		NUR 1202 Pathophysiology	4	(Coop #4)		ENG 1350 Intermediate Writing	4
		PCL 1306 Pharmacology I	2			PCL 1307 Pharmacology II	2
		NUR 1306 Child Health Restor.	10			NUR 1308 Adult Health Restor.	10
			16				16

Junior Year 1998–1999

Fall	QH	Winter	QH	Spring	QH	Summer	QH
PHL 1165 Moral Problems/Med	4	(Coop #5)		ECN 1130 Medical Economics	4	(Coop #6)	
SOC 1320 Statistical Analysis I	4			NUR 1502 Intro to Research	4		
NUR 1408 Mental Health	7			NUR 1406 Healthy Communities	7		
	15				15		

Senior Year 1999–2000

Fall	QH	Winter	QH	Spring	QH	Summer	QH
(Coop #7)		NUR 1508 Mgmt & Leading	6	NUR 1507 Nursing Practicum	6		
		Humanities Elective	4	General Elective	4		
		Computer Elective	4	General Elective	4		
		History Elective	4	General Elective	4		
			18		18		

Total QH = 176

* For students entering/re-entering Fall, 1995.

173

take their first clinical courses, Promoting Healthy Childbearing and Childrearing and Promoting Healthy Adulthood and Aging. This sequence of courses was designed to introduce the students to the nursing model of care based on health promotion/disease prevention and health restoration/health maintenance. The courses are health oriented with a developmental approach, starting with the pregnant woman and family seeking prenatal care as an entry point into the health care system. Promoting Healthy Childbearing and Childrearing is an eight-credit course comprising 5 lecture hours and 9 clinical hours per week. The clinical experience is an 8-hour day in the community with the extra hour accumulated over the quarter to be used for a community-based clinical project. Students are placed in ob/gyn clinics, prenatal classes, and teen parenting classes; make visits with the public health nurse and the home care nurse; and have ultrasound observations of the developing fetus. The students also learn by spending time in Women, Infants, and Children (WIC) offices, well child clinics, with school nurses, in early intervention and early childhood education programs, as well as nursery schools.

The second clinical course, Promoting Healthy Adulthood and Aging, follows the developmental, life-span sequence from young adulthood through the frail elderly years. This clinical course continues to build on the nursing concepts of risk identification, disease prevention, and health maintenance. It is an eight-credit course comprising 5 hours of didactic information and 9 clinical hours weekly. The clinical component of the course is split into one 4-hour community-based experience and one 4-hour clinical experience in a long-term or rehabilitative setting. The extra weekly clinical hour is used for a community-based project. Students interface with adults wherever adults are seeking health care or health information in the community such as primary health care in a clinic setting, occupational health care sites, home care, HIV outreach programs, drug rehabilitation centers, family and women's shelters, and Alcoholics Anonymous meetings. The clinical experience in a long-term or rehabilitative setting introduces students to health care that occurs in an institutional setting while continuing to focus on the nursing care model of primary care and health maintenance. It provides the students with an opportunity to practice nursing skills in a nonintensive, crisis-oriented setting. One important feature of this dual community/long-term care setting is that students see firsthand the end result of preventable conditions. For example, while caring for a patient in the community with hypertension, students are able to care for patients who have suffered strokes as a result of uncontrolled hypertension. This reality becomes a powerful motivator for preventive nursing care.

Because students are spread out in a number of settings, the most essential and defining part of the clinical experience is the pre- and/or postconference. These group experiences are designed so that students share their learning experiences, impressions, and insights. It is within these clinical conferences that the role of the nursing faculty becomes paramount. While community faculty are often in attendance, it is the responsibility of the nursing faculty member to make clear to the nursing students the interface between health care and nursing care. All that the students have observed, experienced, or questioned must be framed within the nursing model, "How can I, as a nurse, make a difference in this situation?"

It is not unusual to have a bewildered student recount a clinical experience such as a home visit to a 16-year-old, single mother of one-month-old twins, who, at age 5, immigrated with her family from Southeast Asia. It is up to the nursing faculty member to identify issues and facilitate discussion on appropriate nursing interventions such as, culturally appropriate family and parenting expectations, support systems for the young mother, feeding, clothing, safety, and environmental concerns for the infants, along with the more obvious primary health care expectations.

Community partners are invited to attend the students' clinical conferences. This provides an opportunity for nursing faculty to teach community health care professionals about the role and discipline of nursing. The presence of community partners models for the students and the interdisciplinary team approach is so essential in community-based primary care. In fact, community faculty members who participate in the clinical conferences often enhance student learning by bringing their knowledge of community members and support systems to the discussions.

Student Assignments

The Northeastern University curriculum is designed to capitalize on the students' own knowledge of families and health. Students have experienced family life and are aware of their own health and health-seeking behaviors. Students are encouraged to reflect on their own circumstances and then transfer this knowledge and understanding of self-care to care of another, to appreciate that knowledge of the familiar can be used to understand the unknown.

Students are assigned to do a weekly journal. By keeping a weekly journal, students engage in self-reflection that helps them identify their own beliefs and then determine how this new self-awareness will affect their practice of nursing. Responses to weekly reading assignments become part of the students' journal. The weekly readings cover such things as an empowering work and clinical practice environment, developing a self-health promotion plan, recounting a home visit made in the past and contrasting their home with another, analyzing personal risk factors, and looking at stressful situations and burnout factors. The weekly journal assignment provides an opportunity for students to synthesize knowledge as they progress through their experiences.

Students are introduced to their community through a tour of the neighborhood. They are expected to record their first impressions by completing an environmental survey. They must also do a key informant interview with a selected member of the community. By sharing their observations and information, students learn that there are many ways to view a situation and multiple realities within the same community. Students must complete a family assessment paper as well as a cultural assessment on patients of their choosing which allows a more in-depth look at community members. In addition to these assignments, students keep a log of patient encounters and are expected to do selected nursing care plans.

Because education is such an important part of nursing, students are expected to do a teaching-learning project based on teaching and learning precepts. Students are paired and identify a group within the community to teach. With group input, the students decide what the learning needs are, identify a teaching plan, and choose methodologies appropriate for the group. The design, implementation, and evaluation of the project follows a grant proposal model with appropriate budgeting for student time and materials.

STUDENT PROFESSIONAL DEVELOPMENT

When compared with a hospital or institutional environment, the dynamics of working in a community are very different. Nurses are no longer "on their own turf" but are invited guests into patients' homes. Nurses become acquainted with the neighborhood children through their schools and day cares. Nurses work with adults in their workplace and in community agencies. Health care becomes a partnership. The nurse and the patient and family enter into a negotiation, share in the decision making, and reach mutually agreed-on goals in the delivery of appropriate health and nursing care.

Teaching professional identity and professional behavior takes on new meaning when nursing students learn in the community. Traditionally, nurses were readily identified by extrinsic trappings, a uniform, a cap, a stethoscope. In the community, where the nurse is not so easily identified, an intrinsic knowledge of one's professional identity is what matters. Caring interactions with the patient as well as knowledgeable, skillful delivery of nursing care are what the patient and community appreciate and remember. To help the students develop a professional demeanor and appearance, Northeastern University has a dress code that prohibits casual clothing such as jeans, T-shirts, sneakers, and other "student" type attire. Men must were ties. This kind of professional responsibility has made a difference in how the students perceive themselves and how others interact with them.

Learning and working in the community forces the nursing student to appreciate the part that health care plays in patients' lives. As health care providers, nurses often focus on health care to the exclusion of other critical issues that affect patients. By working and learning in the community, the nurse begins to understand how a patient prioritizes important concerns—family, school, work, safety, food, and recreation. For many people, health care is not a top priority. Students learn that patients must provide for food, housing, and safety before they can pay attention to health care.

WHAT IS AHEAD

Having adopted a community-based model of nursing education, the faculty at Northeastern University's College of Nursing are mindful that our curriculum will need to continue to evolve as we move forward. One of the mainstays of our philosophy is to teach students and ourselves to regard change as the status quo, not only to anticipate change but take advantage of it in pursuit of our goals of quality patient care.

REFERENCES

Matteson, P. (Ed.). (1995). *Teaching nursing in the neighborhoods. The Northeastern University Model.* New York: Springer.

SECTION V

Implementation Projects in Nursing Programs

"Ideas That Work"

14

A Home Health Lab

Simulated Home Visits as Part of a College Nursing Lab

Mary C. Capozzi
Heather Reece-Tillack
Elizabeth Windstein

THE HOME HEALTH DILEMMA

Attempting to incorporate home health care into an associate degree nursing program is a major challenge for nursing faculty. Time constraints for clinical experience make it imperative that every learning opportunity be highly beneficial. Since faculty members cannot be in every community setting with their students, we have brought the "community" into our nursing laboratory. This chapter shows how one ADN program prepared first-year nursing students with basic community health skills through initial "home visits" to care for eight "patients" in their nursing lab.

DEVELOPING A HOME HEALTH CARE EXPERIENCE

We hired a nurse with a master's degree in community health and employed part-time by Finger Lakes Visiting Nurse Service (FLVNS) to instruct students both in the laboratory and during the follow-up agency experience. Each week throughout the semester, a different group of eight to nine students, one from each medical-surgical clinical group meets for four hours in the nursing laboratory, instead of reporting to their assigned hospital. Both the rotation of students into the lab and the development and correction of the students' written assignment is carried out by a full-time faculty member with a master's degree in community health. Overload compensation was provided for this role.

Home Health Care Laboratory

During the first part of the four-hour lab, the part-time home care nursing instructor discussed home health theory, documentation, treatment modalities, and the various settings in which nurses practice outside acute care hospitals. Students are encouraged to share their previous home care experiences, be they personal or work related.

The second part of the four-hour lab consisted of eight simulated home visits to a variety of clients and their families. The nursing laboratory is converted into a small community, each cubicle representing a different home setting. Home care scenarios are role-played in the nursing lab to provide a realistic home visit. The nursing students assume the role of the client, family/caregiver, home care nurse, or observer. The scenarios represent a cross-section of home care cases, enabling the student nurse to practice technical, teaching, assessment, and intervention skills. The role-playing scenarios provide a nonthreatening environment for students to learn and practice new skills with the support of their peers. Scenarios can be modified to include any diagnosis, home situation, or treatment. This model lab is most effective for groups of 6 to 10 students who are beginning their home care clinical experience. The lab experience prepares students for the following day when they affiliate at a home health agency and participate in actual home visits with an agency nurse.

When possible, the clients' diagnoses, nursing needs, and treatments are coordinated with the students' medical-surgical curriculum. Home health lab objective are met through the active participation of each student in a home visit role-playing scenario. Eight home care scenarios have been developed incorporating the patient's medical record, physician's orders, treatments, and medications, as needed, for reference.

Socioeconomic and psychosocial profiles are also included. With each home visit, one student is assigned to the role of the client and another to the role of family or significant other. To encourage professional collaboration with these home care problems, two nursing students are assigned to the role of visiting nurses. Students complete several nursing procedures in each scenario. The remaining students are assigned to coach, observe, and assist the "home care nurses" with unfamiliar procedures or suggest interventions to help with a family problem.

The home care scenario is presented to the group. The students assigned to role-play receive cue cards, which include a description of the coping level and personality traits of the family and patient. Students are encouraged to "ham up" their roles allowing for more spontaneous reactions.

The setting for each lab scenario is tailored to the client's living situation. During each visit, a problem is presented that requires critical thinking and action by the nurse. The clients and their families have health problems common to many home care clients. Complicating the situations are secondary medical diagnoses (e.g., poor vision) and dysfunctional family situations. The students, assigned to the role of visiting nurses, complete various assessments and patient care procedures with an emphasis on teaching the client and the family. Empowering the client and family to assume as many self-care activities as possible is encouraged in the lab. Students often see this as a different approach from that used for clients and families in the hospital. The faculty acts as facilitator, resource, and guide to the students during these assessments, interactions, and assigned procedures. Students, who are either observing or role-playing, are free to ask questions or offer comments throughout the simulated home visit. After each scenario, the group discusses the situation and develops nursing diagnoses, short- and long-term goals, and related nursing interventions.

HOME CARE SCENARIOS

Preparation

Preparation of the nursing lab includes setting up cubicles to represent the clients' homes as described in the scenarios. Props and special effects enhance each scene. Medical mannequins are used for invasive procedures that are not feasible to perform on a student. Adjoining cubicles can be used in these scenarios so the medical mannequin can be in one bed and the student role-playing the client in the other; or the student can sit at the head of the bed of the mannequin. Reference drug books and nursing procedure manuals are available for students. To use space more efficiently, each scenario's props and equipment are stored in a labeled box. These are then placed on a cart and wheeled into each cubicle to set up and to take down.

Guidelines

The following guidelines are used for each scenario:

1. Pass out cue cards to students, describing their roles:
   - 1 client card.
   - 2–3 nurse cards.
   - 1 caregiver/family card.
2. Read or have a student read the family/social data card and the cue cards.
3. The students then role-play the scenario. Cue and direct as needed.
4. Each scenario can vary in length from 10 to 30 minutes, depending on how many nursing interventions are performed and how much discussion is generated.
5. After each scenario, discuss nursing diagnoses, interventions, and plans for the next home visit.
6. Switch roles for the next visits until all students have had the opportunity to be the client, caregiver/family, and nurse.

Cue Card Format

1. *Client Card*—Gives information about the client.
   You are:
   Health Hx:
   Problems:
2. *Nurse Card*—Gives information and direction to the nurse.
   You are the visiting nurse for:
   Medical Dx:
   MD Orders:
   Nursing instructions for assessments and treatments:
   (Two to three nurse cards may be distributed depending on how complicated the case is and to enable all students to have an opportunity to act as the nurse.)

3. *Caregiver/Family Card*—Gives information about the caregiver.

    You are:

    Health Hx:

    Problems:

4. *Family/Social Data Card*—Gives information about the client's family and support system, living arrangements, and coping status, which contributes to the care plan.

5. *Skills Card*—Describes educational opportunities in each scenario.

    A. Technical.

    B. Assessment.

    C. Teaching.

6. *Equipment Card*—Describes what is needed for each scenario.

    A. Scene.

    B. Props.

    C. Equipment.

Client with Diabetes

Scenario 1: Family/Social Data Card

Family/Support System: The client Joan Rogers, a former store clerk and homemaker, is 68 years old, has insulin-dependent diabetes, poor vision, and a slow-healing foot sore. She is cared for by her 73-year-old husband Fred, a retired grocery store manager, who has poor vision and arthritic knees. Since Joan's discharge from the hospital, he has been filling her insulin syringes, helping her check her blood glucose level, preparing her meals, and generally waiting on her, due to her limited mobility and poor vision. Their daughter Glenda is living with them temporarily, while undergoing a divorce. She works days.

Living Arrangements: The Rogers live in a two-story older home with the bathroom and bedrooms upstairs. Joan has not been downstairs since her hospital discharge one week ago.

Coping Status: Joan had always been the active caretaker in the family. Since her discharge from the hospital one week ago, she has become demanding of her husband, frustrated with having to stay upstairs in her bedroom to be near the bathroom and worried about her husband drawing up the insulin and overdoing it going up and down the stairs so much.

Fred is getting worn out caring for his wife, which he does willingly and without complaint. He is anxious about doing everything correctly.

Glenda is a loving daughter, but overwhelmed with her marital problems and works long hours to keep her mind occupied.

Scenario 1: Client Card

You Are: Joan Rogers, 68 years old

Health Hx: Insulin-Dependent Diabetic for two years, bilateral cataracts, diabetic ulcer right lateral foot. Recently discharged from hospital after treatment for elevated blood sugar and nonhealing foot ulcer.

Problems

1. Foot ulcer requires daily dressing change which you can't do.
2. Blood glucose still elevated some days.
3. Feeling tired and worthless being in bedroom all day.
4. Worried about loss of role and independence.
5. Worried about husband doing too much and his accuracy in preparing your insulin and glucometer checks because of his poor vision.

Props

Cataract glasses

Scenario 1: Caregiver/Family Card

You Are: Fred Rogers, 73 years old, husband of the client

Health Hx: Tunnel vision and arthritis in both knees.

Problems

1. Nervous about doing dressing change.
2. Not sure if you are drawing up insulin accurately and doing glucometer correctly.
3. The arthritis in your knees is acting up because of all the stair climbing.
4. Worried about your wife's change in behavior from being in control to being tired, demanding, discouraged.

Props

Tunnel vision glasses

Scenario 1: Nurse Card

You Are the Visiting Nurse for: Joan Rogers, 68 years old

Medical Dx:

1. IDDM.
2. Diabetic Ulcer R lateral foot.
3. HTN.
4. Bilateral Cataracts.

MD Orders Include: NPH insulin 20 units SQ qAM, FBS with glucometer daily, 2000 ADA diet. Wound Care: QD irrigate with normal saline, wet to dry NS dressing, wrap with kerlex, limit ambulation until next appointment. Wound Culture.

Nursing Assessments and Interventions

1. Wound care, do dressing, instruct husband, assess his ability to do dressing.
2. Diabetic regime: observe husband's ability to prepare insulin, use glucometer, assess understanding of diet and hypo/hyperglycemia.
3. Assess family's coping mechanisms and ability to do care.

Scenario 1: Skills Card

Technical

Handwashing, vital signs, insulin preparation, glucometer readings, wet to dry dressing change, universal precautions.

Teaching

Diabetic regime, wound care.

Assessment

Diabetic status, wound status, visual acuity, ability to do care, mobility impairment, coping status.

Scenario 1: Supply Card

Scene: Client's bedroom

Props

1. Glasses smeared with petroleum jelly to represent cataracts.
2. Glasses with lenses covered except for small holes to represent tunnel vision.
3. Electric cord across room as a safety hazard.
4. Afghan and pillow on chair.
5. Name tags identifying roles.
6. Furnishings: two chairs, bed, table.

Supplies

Nursing Bag

    Blood pressure cuff

    Stethoscope

    Thermometer

    Handwashing supplies

    Sharps container

Dressing Change
  2 pair exam gloves
  2 packs 4 × 4 gauze sponges
  Bottle of normal saline
  Tape
  Culture Swab
Insulin Teaching
  Insulin syringes (2 sizes low and high dose)
  Insulin bottle
  Alcohol swabs
  Glucometer
Visual Assessment
  Magnifier aid for syringe
  Newspaper
  Culture swab

Client with BKA

Scenario 2: Family/Social Data Card

Family/Support System: The client, Samuel Jones, is a 65-year-old retired policeman who recently had a BKA. He cares for himself with assistance from a
neighbor, Grace, and a HHA.

Living Arrangements: Mr. Jones lives alone in a small, downstairs apartment.

Coping Status: Mr. Jones is very independent, despite health problems. He is active and drove his own car until this surgery. He is anxious to get driving again.
He is pleasant and has a great attitude.
  Grace is Sam's neighbor who stops by daily to check on him and is anxious
to help.

Scenario 2: Client Card

You Are: Sam Jones, 65 years old

Health Hx: Right BKA with open incision, Hx HTN, colostomy 2o to Ca of
colon 1992, IDDM—under control, self-care.

Problems

1. Requires assistance with dressing change.
2. Ostomy bag has been leaking.
3. Decreased mobility.
4. Learning to use crutches.
5. Decreased independence.

Props

Baseball cap

Scenario 2: Caregiver/Family Card

You Are: Grace, Sam's upstairs neighbor, 57 years old, lives alone.

Health Hx: None significant.

Problems

1. Wants to assist Sam with dressing change.

2. Has worked as an aide in the past; wants to learn how to change dressing.

Scenario 2: Nurse Card

You Are the Visiting Nurse for: Sam Jones, 65 years old, retired policeman.

Medical Hx:

1. Right BKA with draining incision.
2. IDDM.
3. Colostomy 2o to colon CA 1992.

MD Orders Include:

Wound care qd, wet to dry NS dressing on right stump, wrap with ace. Physical therapy, occupational therapy, evaluate and Tx, ambulate with crutches.

Nursing Assessments and Interventions

1. Wound care as ordered, wrap stump.
2. Assess colostomy function, change ostomy bag.
3. Supervise crutch walking.
4. Evaluate ability to do ADLs.
5. Assess diabetic status.

Scenario 2: Skills Card

Technical

Handwashing, dressing change, stump wrap, use of crutches, ostomy bag change.

Teaching

Wound care, dressing change, use of crutches.

Assessment

Wound status, ostomy bag, safety, ability to ambulate.

Scenario 2: Supply Card

Scene: Client's bedroom, table, 2 hospital beds (one with mannequin)

Props

1. Baseball cap
2. Medical mannequin with colostomy and right BKA

Supplies

Nursing Bag
   Blood pressure cuff
   Stethoscope

Dressing Change
   Exam gloves
   2 packs 4 × 4 gauze sponges
   Bottle of normal saline
   4" × 6" Ace bandage
   Tape

Colostomy
   Variety of colostomy appliances
   Towels

Ambulate
   Crutches

HEALTH AGENCY VISIT

Day two consists of a four-hour block of time during which the student is paired with a nurse from a home health agency. During this time, the nurse and the student make actual home visits. The role of our faculty member at the agency is to assist the agency with assigning students. She informs the nurses of the students' abilities to perform various interventions within the home and reviews charts for nursing interventions that the students could participate in. She works with the agency's staff educator to give students a brief orientation. The students review charts with the guidance of the nursing instructor while the visiting nurse prepares for the home visit. Students are instructed to observe and participate, when possible, in the assessment and treatments that are provided during the home visit. Practical needs of the client are identified as well as any other home health services that are being utilized. The faculty member may also make home visits to a select group of patients with a student.

Students are encouraged to recognize the importance of discharge planning and its effects on the client's transition from the hospital to the home. The interaction between the visiting nurse and the student allows the student to recognize the uniqueness of each home care visit. Observing and assisting the visiting nurse provide the student with a different approach to nursing than that observed in the hospital setting. The home health experience familiarizes the student with home care as an important facet of health care today.

LEARNING OUTCOMES

Goals for the Home Health Lab include:

1. Students will collaborate with each other while developing a plan of care and/or carrying out a procedure.
2. Students will be able to identify challenges that are presented with providing care in a community setting.
3. Students will be able to develop a teaching plan for a client and/or the client's family.
4. Students will demonstrate empathy for the client and/or family through role-playing.
5. Students will demonstrate the ability to perform assessments and assigned treatments with minimal guidance.

WRITTEN ASSIGNMENT

A clinical assignment has been developed to help the student integrate the essentials of home care with the nursing process. One home visit is critically evaluated after the home care experience. The assignment requires the student to review information in the patient record including doctor's orders, medications, and any support services used or needed by the patient or family. The student is required to describe what assessments are done and what information is obtained along with identifying equipment and supplies that are utilized during the visit. Physical, psychosocial, economic, and cultural aspects that influence patient care are incorporated into the assignment. After gathering this information, the student writes one nursing diagnosis related to the home health care needs of the patient and/or the family. The student then writes a goal and three nursing interventions related to the nursing diagnosis.

STUDENT EVALUATIONS

Written evaluations are done at the end of the second day. As indicted by the following comments, the students found the experience beneficial:

- "Great opportunity to practice competencies."
- "I never considered home care, but I loved it."
- "I'm beginning to understand the benefits of home care."
- "Good preparation for clinical."

SUMMARY

Home health nursing concepts are taught in the freshman year through a home health lab. This lab provides a controlled and efficient setting for a variety of simulated home visits. As a result, students expand their awareness of home care and are better prepared for their role in community nursing.

15

Designing, Implementing, and Evaluating a Transition Course

Moving Registered Nurses from Acute Care to Home Care

Geraldine C. Colombraro

Managed care has begun to penetrate the New York metropolitan area, making slow but steady progress. As hospitals positioned themselves for managed care, acute care nurses expressed increasing concern not only about their job security but also about deteriorating working conditions that were seriously compromised by staffing patterns that characteristically used fewer RNs and more unlicensed assistive personnel. As an American Nurses Credentialling Center's Commission on Accreditation approved provider of continuing education in nursing, the Center for Continuing Education in Nursing and Health Care provides approximately 100 continuing education activities to thousands of nurses each year and is recognized as a valuable professional resource in the community. In 1994, the Center began to receive calls from nurses in acute care settings throughout the metropolitan area asking if we offered a course to help them make the move into home care. Although the Nurse Refresher course was available, a "transitions" course was not something the Center had ever offered. Throughout 1994, we explored the possibilities of developing such a course with colleagues both within the Lienhard School of Nursing and in a variety of home care agencies. Because of our confidence in the project's eventual success, we began to collect names and addresses from callers who were potential participants.

Two events early in 1995 made the development of a transitions course a reality. The volume of interested callers increased dramatically, and the

New York State Nurses Association (NYSNA) approached the Lienhard School of Nursing, Pace University, to discuss jointly offering this course. Planning began in earnest through the spring 1995 semester after a meeting I attended with Elizabeth Carter, Deputy Executive Director of NYSNA; Carolyn McCullough, NYSNA's Director of Economic and General Welfare; and Dean Harriet Feldman of Lienhard.

We decided to use our highly successful Nurse Refresher course as a model for the development of the transitions course. Participants would spend 5 full days over an 8-week period at Pace University for didactic presentations and discussions. They would also spend 40 hours in a home care agency, working with RNs in patients' homes. Although we knew of one other provider in our area who was offering a classroom-only transitions course, it was our belief that to do so would be like offering a refresher course without any hospital experience. Our philosophy was that mandatory clinical experience would complement and enhance the classroom portion of the Pace transitions course, making the participants more marketable in today's competitive job market. Finding clinical agencies to work with us in this first effort was, perhaps, the most difficult part of the planning process. Through contacts in home care, the Center was able to identify three agencies that agreed to collaborate with the Center to implement the course in the fall of 1995. Quite understandably, the home care agencies were concerned about the entry requirements for the course. At a planning meeting, the agencies defined the entry requirements that they felt were necessary, including an active New York State RN license, the state-mandated course "Training in Barrier Precautions and Infection Control Measures," health clearance, and malpractice insurance. We also included "current acute care experience" as a requirement. After much discussion, the agencies felt they did not want to limit this experience to a specific area, nor did they feel it would be helpful to specify staff versus supervisory experience or what degree (e.g., BSN) was needed. The agencies wanted the flexibility to accept or refuse a candidate based on total qualifications rather than an arbitrary constraint. It was agreed that participants would be interviewed by the home care agency first; applicants accepted by the agency for the clinical component of the course were then accepted by Pace for the classroom component.

The course was marketed by direct mail and by articles in NYSNA's monthly newsletters and *Nursing Spectrum*. Because the Center had been collecting names for over a year, we already had a database of names and addresses of nurses interested in a transitions course. The first NYSNA article ran in the July 1995 newsletter, resulting in hundreds of additional calls to the Center by interested nurses. The information about the course was mailed to all the nurses on our mailing list as well as all callers beginning in July 1995. We had determined that this first course would be a pilot limited to 24 nurses; it was fully enrolled by the beginning of September 1995.

In determining the classroom content for the transitions course, we once again followed the Nurse Refresher model: We asked the home care agencies we were working with what they would want a nurse to know about home care to get a job with their agency. This highly pragmatic approach helped us design a curriculum that focused on the requisite knowledge, skills, and abilities for a nurse working in a home care setting (see Table 15–1 for Classroom Objectives).

A Pace University faculty member, Dr. Ilse Leeser, RN, FNP, volunteered to work with the Center to teach two days of the didactic portion of the course: the introduction to home care and physical assessment in the home. Two clinical agencies volunteered to teach an additional two days: reimbursement and documentation, and clinical issues in home care. Finally, on the fifth day, presenters included a nurse attorney at address legal aspects of home care, Dr. Leeser on ethics in home care, and two nurse recruiters from a home care agency to discuss career opportunities in home care. This team approach would expose participants to several experts, each of whom would provide a unique perspective about home care.

The clinical agencies agreed that they would offer the nurses varied home care experiences—but in different ways, depending on the resources available in each agency. One agency hired a clinical instructor to work with the transitions participants. Another agency partnered each participant with an RN. The third agency combined these approaches. Each method had both strengths and weaknesses, and participants were always encouraged to discuss their learning needs with the agencies.

An interesting aspect of the clinical experience was whether the participants would be allowed to do hands-on care, or would be limited purely to observation. Two of the three agencies restricted the experience to observation only, while the third agency allowed supervised hands-on care. Participants were told what their experiences would be when they interviewed with the agency, so their expectations were clear before they registered for the course. In all agencies, participants were exposed to intake visits, interdisciplinary team meetings, and educational sessions as

Table 15–1
Transition from Acute Care to
Home Care Classroom Objectives

Day One: Overview of Home Care

1. Recognize the roles and responsibilities of the RN in the home care setting.
2. Understand and analyze the functions of the interdisciplinary health care team in meeting the needs of the patient/family in the home care setting.
3. Analyze the role of the RN in the coordination of services and long-term discharge planning.
4. Understand the application of the nursing process through home visits.

Day Two: Operational Aspects of Home Care

1. Define case management.
2. Differentiate between case management and managed care.
3. Identify the role of the RN in managed care.
4. Identify the role of the case manager in managed care.
5. Identify methods of reimbursement in home care.
6. Understand the basic concepts of criteria and coverage in home care.
7. Identify the nurse's role in determining financial coverage and services needed.
8. Identify basic principles of reimbursement in home care.
9. Discuss parts of the home care record.
10. Discuss how home care nursing standards and scope influence documentation.
11. Discuss how insurance criteria affect documentation.

Day Three: Clinical Issues in Home Care

1. Discuss home infusion programs.
2. Discuss the role of the home care nurse in providing home infusion therapies and coordination of home care services.
3. Describe rehabilitation services and referral patterns in home care.
4. Identify fundamental home care assessment skills for rehabilitation needs at home.
5. Discuss the uses of rehabilitation equipment in the home.
6. Discuss the physiology of the skin and the pathophysiology of wounds.
7. Identify and describe the importance of home care standards of clinical management for wound care.
8. Recognize and discuss the basic components of an effective teaching plan.
9. Outline admission and discharge criteria.
10. Recognize environmental factors that increase the spread of pathogenic organisms.
11. Plan strategies to prevent the spread of pathogenic organisms in the home.
12. Identify the role of the nurse in medication management at home.
13. Identify three reasons for patient nonadherence to medication regimen.
14. Identify measures to improve adherence to medication schedule.
15. Describe potential barriers to patient/family learning.
16. Identify ways to improve patient/family teaching.

Table 15–1 (Continued)

Day Four: Overview of Physical Assessment in the Home Care Setting

1. Understand the principles of physical assessment in the home care setting.
2. Use appropriate interviewing skills to elicit a health history from individuals of various ages and cultures.
3. Demonstrate a systematic approach to health assessment.
4. Incorporate developmental and cultural components of the individual/family in interpreting data gathered from clinical assessment.
5. Identify deviations from normal physical assessment findings.

Day Five

A. Legal and Ethical Issues in Home Care

1. Discuss hospital DNR order, health care proxy, and living wills in the home care setting.
2. Discuss violations of federal Medicare, fraud, and abuse statutes in home care.
3. Discuss the federal antireferral law in home care.
4. Discuss professional misconduct in home care.
5. Discuss elder abuse in home care.
6. Analyze problems in home care involving patient, family and/or nurses's decision making that pose ethical dilemmas; explore viable options in dealing with these ethical considerations in the home care setting.

B. Career Opportunities

1. Review understanding of home care options versus hospital nursing.
2. Identify positions that are currently available in home care.
3. Identify requirements for positions.
4. Discuss how to prepare a professional resume.
5. Discuss how to use a "head hunter."
6. Discuss how to read and respond to ads.
7. Discuss how to compose an appropriate cover letter.
8. Discuss how to present/conduct yourself during the interview.

Note: Copyright 1996. Pace University. Reprinted with permission.

available (see Table 15–2 for Clinical Objectives). On the first day of class, I listened carefully as participants described their current positions, years of experience, and reasons for taking this course. What was striking was the vast amount of acute care experience that each participant brought to the transitions course. Clinical experiences centered around ICU, CCU, OR, ER, Labor and Delivery, with an average of at least 20 years acute care experience per participant. These nurses were discouraged and angry with what they saw happening in acute care. One nurse described how her hospital's downsizing required her to float to different

Table 15–2
Transition from Acute Care to Home Care: Clinical Objectives

1. General Goal: Provide participants with a broad overview of the role of the RN in home care.
2. Differentiate between licensed and certified home care agencies.
3. Observe the entire admission process for a minimum of 2 or 3 home care patients including (but not necessarily limited to):
   a. Referral on intake.
   b. Determination of acceptance (or denial).
   c. First visit (major responsibility).
   d. Determination of appropriate services to be given.
   e. Determination of frequency of visits.
4. Within the context of revisits, observe/implement the plan of care for as broad a range of patients as possible, such as:
   a. Cardiac patient.
   b. Diabetic patient.
   c. COPD patient.
   d. Wound and skin care.
   e. New baby/mother.
   f. Ventilators.
   g. IV therapy.
   h. Rehab.
   i. Pediatrics.
   j. Hospice.
   k. Placement and supervision of HHAs and/or PCAs.
5. Observe high tech in the home, as available.
6. Increase knowledge and skills concerning documentation and paperwork for home care, including "practice" nursing notes and skilled observations.
7. Discuss the application of interdisciplinary case management in the home, including how to take a patient report, write it up, and how to speak to insurance case managers.

Note: Copyright 1996. Pace University. Reprinted with permission.

units all over the house; she ended her lament with, "I am at wit's end!" Another nurse echoed her dismay, stressing, "I am not happy with the shift away from the patient." In fact, most nurses expected that home care would enable them to spend more time with patients, deal with patients on a personal level, do more patient teaching, and simply have more patient contact than the acute care setting allowed them.

Most participants insisted they had no intention of moving into home care immediately after completing this course. They saw it, instead, as an opportunity to make themselves more marketable and to prepare themselves for the future "just in case." Several nurses indicated they either were in a home care/community health master's program or would be reentering higher education to complete their baccalaureate in nursing or earn a master's in nursing in home care/community health nursing. Most indicated that they wanted either to be prepared for whatever happened or to explore home care as a positive step in their nursing careers.

When the participants met for the second week of class, differences in the home care agencies became evident as participants discussed what they had seen or done in the previous week. One participant was distressed that she had not seen certain types of patients, and she was advised to speak with the home care agency to actively seek out these experiences. Hearing what other participants were seeing or doing was useful to all of them. Each week, the instructor was instrumental in helping participants link what they were learning in the classroom to what they were seeing in patients' homes.

All participants were required to complete 40 hours of clinical before the last day of class. Participants contracted with the home care agency to determine how they would meet this requirement. Some participants worked 5, eight-hour days; others worked 10, four-hour blocks of time. One agency actually called specific participants when it accepted patients with a particular health problem that the participant had expressed interest in. Many participants expected to work evenings or weekends, which could not be arranged by the home care agencies. Because the course was a major commitment of time, participants needed to clear time from their schedules to complete the clinical requirement.

Evaluation was conducted at many different levels. Participants evaluated the classroom component on a weekly basis; the home care agencies did clinical evaluations at the end of the clinical experience; faculty who taught the course, both in the classroom and in clinical, also evaluated it. Finally, Dr. Leeser and I met all the home care agency representatives to discuss the evaluations and plan for the next course.

Student evaluations of both the classroom and the clinical experiences were overwhelmingly positive, although several interesting findings should be noted here. The participants truly relished the client-centered approach that home care requires and repeatedly emphasized that the best experience was "spending time with patients again." Most participants were surprised with how much the home care nurse was required to know, including adult, maternal-child, and pediatric care, high-tech IV therapy, wound care, hospice care—and, of course, paperwork! Several participants expressed frustration with "wasted time" necessitated by organizing visits for the day or making phone calls, but after further discussion among the group, determined that the perceived lack of organization may have simply been an indication that home care nurses work at a different pace than acute care nurses.

The cost of the course was an issue for a number of participants, who indicated that they found it to be expensive. The classroom fee was $399, and the clinical fee was $399; participants received a total of 73 hours of instruction. After discussion among the group, it was determined that those health care agencies represented by NYSNA not only reimbursed their nurses for this course, but they also gave them time off from their acute care job to attend both classroom and clinical. Some other hospitals reimbursed the nurses for all or part of this course, while some hospitals did not reimburse the nurses because this course did not help them perform their acute care job better.

The participants found that cultural aspects of care were critically important in home care. As one ICU nurse shared, "When I have a patient in the ICU, it almost doesn't matter what his culture is. But in the home, culture really comes through and *I had to change* to accommodate the patient's needs." One participant shared that she had lived in the Bronx all her life, but never knew about all its different neighborhoods until she started making home visits. None of the participants expressed a desire to make the change to a home care position immediately, primarily because salaries are much lower in home care than acute care. However, many participants expressed interest in finding a part-time position in home care to complement their acute care position. As one participant enthusiastically said in summary, "I'm more convinced that this is what I want to do than ever!"

The home care agencies each evaluated the participant's clinical experiences using their own tools. Once again, the participant's evaluations were quite positive. In one agency, participants recommended either using a smaller group or hiring another instructor due to a high participant/instructor ratio. This agency agreed to reduce the number of participants they accepted for the next course. In another agency, participants reported they observed nurses doing too much supervision of home health aides versus actual patient care; this agency agreed to try to expand the types of experiences their participants had. And in the third agency, participants were exposed to a wide variety of cases and experiences, which they evaluated very positively. Some participants were asked if they would recommend this course to a friend, and they indicated that they would.

The pilot course ended in November, and an evaluation/planning meeting was held in early December. All the clinical agencies were represented, as were Dr. Leeser and myself; evaluation data were shared by all parties. From Pace's perspective, the course was a success. The classroom evaluations were positive, and the financial revenue/expenditure ratio was strong. We also received several phone inquiries from other home care agencies interested in participating as a site the next time the course was offered, so that the course could be expanded as we originally envisioned. Representatives from these new sites were invited to attend this meeting so that they could learn about the course firsthand. All agreed that this meeting was invaluable, both in evaluating the previous semester and planning for the next semester.

The course was offered a second time in the spring of 1996, with 30 participants in 10 different home care agencies. Logistically, working with 10 agencies instead of 3 was considerably more complicated but provided participants with a wealth of choices. Good communication between the staff of the Center and each home care agency was critical. Each agency could take a smaller number of participants, with less drain on their resources. From the classroom perspective, there was no significant difference in having 24 or 30 participants in the room.

From the home care agencies' perspectives, the course was also a success. The agencies were paid directly by the participants for the clinical component of the course, so that the agencies recouped their costs. An interesting finding was that because the participants themselves were so experienced and so skilled, the home care nurses enjoyed working with them and even said that they learned from the participants. Several home care agency representatives said that now that they had participated in this course, they would be more willing to hire a participant even if the person had no home care experience. How does Pace's experience compare to other providers' experiences retraining acute care nurses for home care? Several studies (Keating, 1994; O'Neil & Pennington, 1996; O'Shea, 1994) have identified the need to retrain acute care nurses for home care practice. O'Neil and Pennington described a consortium that was developed in Massachusetts to help nurses move from acute care to home care. They reported that hospitals were able to ease the nurses' transition through flexible hours and financial support. This is similar to our finding that nurses represented by NYSNA were most comfortable participating in this course. They also reported that collaboration with community agencies has facilitated student placement in the undergraduate and graduate departments of the university. We, too, found that several home care agencies have expressed appreciation for the opportunity to collaborate with the university. The agencies have met with program chairpersons to negotiate student placements from our degree programs. Even more exciting, one agency has approached Pace to collaborate on research on outcomes of home care. This is a wonderful opportunity for Pace's graduate students to participate in meaningful research for their theses.

SUMMARY

The transition course has proven a win-win-win opportunity for Pace, for the home care agencies, and for the participants. Participants are truly prepared to work in home care settings. Now that a year has gone by since the first group took the transitions course, we are surveying that pilot group to determine how many have actually made this transition. The home care agencies have hired several graduates of the transitions course; however, they were under no obligation to hire any of the participants. The fees from the course paid to the home care agencies covered the costs the agencies incurred. Pace was able to work collaboratively with a wide range of agencies to develop a course desperately needed by the professional community in the tristate area. As managed care penetration increases in our region, we anticipate that the need for this course will increase: Hospitals will close beds and units while home care agencies are providing sign-on bonuses for RNs.

REFERENCES

Keating, S. B. (1994). Hospital nursing care expanding into the home. *Geriatric Nursing, 15*(5), 282–283.

O'Neil, E. S., & Pennington, E. A. (1996). Preparing acute care nurses for community based care. *Nursing and Health Care: Perspectives on Community, 17*(2), 62–65.

O'Shea, A. M. (1994). Transitioning professional nurses into home care: A 6-month mentorship program. *Journal of Home Health Care Practice, 6*(4), 67–72.

16

Preparing Associate Degree Graduates for Immediate Employment in Home Health

Clare T. Garrard

Home health agencies are increasingly being utilized as clinical placement sites by associate degree nursing programs across the country (Noble, Redmond, Williams, & Langley, 1996). While this is a positive clinical experience for the students, the lack of immediate employment following graduation is frustrating. Working collaboratively with a local home health agency, one associate degree nursing program was able to successfully implement a program that prepared new graduates for immediate employment in a home health care agency.

COMMUNITY FOCUS WITHIN THE ASSOCIATE DEGREE CURRICULUM

Shifting health care demographics reflect the trend toward increasing acuity of hospital admissions, early discharge rates, and increased utilization of home health care agencies. In northwest Georgia, local hospitals have reduced the number of registered nurse positions, while increasing the number of assistive personnel. One local home health care agency reports a greater number of RN full-time employees than the local hospitals.

Typically, the home health care agencies in this area require new graduates to have at least one year of acute care experience to be considered for employment. Local nurse recruiters for both acute care and home health care agencies reflect a 20–35 percent turnover annually. As one home health manager from the community explained, "The acute care nurse may not be comfortable with the autonomy or the pace of home health. They stay for about three months, then return to the more comfortable environment of acute care. Those who like this area of nursing stay approximately 7 years." Since orientation for each new hire is estimated to cost between $10,000 and $15,000, the home health administrators would understandably prefer to hire those nurses who have the greatest probability of becoming long-term employees. New graduates who have had significant clinical placement in home health were positioned to become long-term employees.

DEVELOPMENT OF THE PILOT PROJECT

With the changing job market, the associate degree nursing program sought to provide clinical experiences in areas where employment was probable for new graduates. Since the home health agency was eager to provide clinical experience for students, we sought to develop a program that would allow immediate employment for selected new graduates. Having defined this goal, a number of significant barriers became apparent.

Storming the Barriers

Barriers existed within the nursing faculty. To overcome initial resistance to this program, the conceptual framework of the curriculum was revisited. Desired terminal outcomes were identified that reflected competencies, attitudes, and behaviors. Clinical experiences were then matched with the corresponding competencies and behaviors. Although home health care consistently provided a variety of skills and behaviors as well as excellent role models (Kaiser & Rudolph, 1996), faculty clung tenaciously to the belief that only acute care experience would adequately prepare new graduates to function in the "real world." To overcome this barrier, a survey was conducted to determine the frequency with which certain essential skills were encountered in both the acute care and the home health arena. Home health nurses indicated that they were routinely performing catheterization, NG tube placement and enteral feedings, IV therapy, IM and subcutaneous medication administration, care of the ventilator-dependent patient in the home including airway management, dressing changes, and patient teaching. The acute care nurses reported that they were less frequently able to provide these experiences for the students. Faculty who were not experienced in home health agreed to work with home health nurses to determine the suitability of this experience for our students.

Agency Concerns

The home health agency articulated some concerns regarding both clinical placement and immediate employment.

Confidentiality of patient information as well as agency liability were also issues to be addressed. Students were required to pass a clinical skills check-off prior to assignment in home health for clinical experience. All students undergo confidentiality training annually and document that they understand the severity of any breach of confidence. Students signed a waiver releasing the home health nurse from liability during travel and carried school-mandated professional liability insurance. Having surmounted these barriers, the next task was to increase the confidence levels of both faculty and clinical personnel as practitioners and teachers.

Train the Trainers

College faculty worked with agency staff nurses to familiarize themselves with the agency policies and procedures as well as the components of routine home health visits. During these sessions, faculty functioned as novice learners, working toward skill acquisition and mastery (Patterson, 1996). The unfamiliar jargon of home care, documentation, and recertification soon became second nature. The relationship of the clinical liaison to the field nurse and physician's office was clarified. There was an evident emphasis on teaching/learning, identification of goals, and progress toward goal achievement. Simultaneously, the field nurses learned to function as faculty, asking leading questions, demonstrating a procedure, then allowing the faculty member to return the demonstration (Davies, White, Riley, & Twinn, 1996).

The clients were prepared for the students' visits by the faculty and field nurses. In addition, families received written guidelines for student experiences, being assured that the students would be strictly supervised and that the client had the right to refuse to have a student at any time. No refusals were received; in fact, the clients took the students' experiences very seriously, asking the students questions not only about their medications and treatments, but also about the students' reactions to each experience. Clients were very interested in a student's performance on exams pertinent to the client's particular problem (e.g., "Did you do well on the diabetes part of the test? Now, I told you about vision trouble, didn't I?"). These interactions put a very personal face on an impersonal disease, helping the students analyze the impact of chronic disease on everyday life.

Course Outcomes

The conceptual model used for this pilot project combined didactic and clinical experiences through two quarters, culminating in potential employment. During the fifth quarter of the program, students had an opportunity to select a three-week home health clinical experience, in lieu of one medical-surgical rotation. Students were assigned to an agency field nurse, and accompanied that nurse on assigned days. Students were allowed to perform physical assessments, accu-checks, patient teaching, and dressing changes. The same skills were matched by their peers in the hospital setting. These skills were documented in the patient's record and the field nurse cosigned with the student. Faculty participated in at least one home visit with each student during the rotation. Thirty-five students selected this experience.

Preceptorship Experience

During the final quarter of the program, all students participated in a preceptorship experience. A select number of students ($n-15$) chose a preceptorship in home health. This experience entailed a 20-hour classroom component and 160 clinical hours. During the didactic component, students learned to complete the documentation required from admission to discharge, communicate areas of concern to the clinical liaison or MD, and received in-depth training concerning wound protocols, infusion devices, blood transfusions in the home, and other procedures. Following successful completion of an exit examination, students were assigned to a clinical preceptor. Clinical course objectives were reviewed with the preceptor and student. In addition, the student identified at least five clinical objectives to be accomplished during the rotation. The students logged 160 clinical hours with the field nurse, gradually assuming more and more responsibility during each visit. The faculty made at least eight supervisory visits with the student and field nurse. In addition, faculty met with the preceptor and student at midquarter to determine the student's progress toward goal achievement.

Students were required to attend a weekly seminar in which they discussed the roles and responsibilities of the home health nurse, evaluated their progress toward role acquisition, and shared research findings, practical tips, and techniques for dealing with the homebound population. With the permission of the faculty of the college, the administrative team of the agency, and the College Institutional Review Borad, the students conducted a survey of the homebound elderly to determine the extent of depression within this population. The survey also included items relating to services that were desirable in this population such as visiting clergy. As a result of this collaborative effort, a proposal to provide pastoral care to homebound elderly has been initiated by the home health agency.

As the rotation progressed, both the students and the field nurses were pleased and surprised with the students' professional growth and role acquisition. Field nurses were very relaxed and comfortable with the students' performance. Students expressed an improved level of confidence in their performance of nursing skills as well as their ability to problem-solve and think critically. Faculty were also pleased with the students' role acquisition and display of professionalism during this rotation. Critical thinking skills were enhanced through the networking between student, preceptor, faculty, and staff (Martin, 1996).

OUTCOMES FOLLOWING PILOT PROJECT

At the conclusion of the terminal quarter, evaluative comments were solicited from the faculty, students, preceptors, and clients. Graduates found the experience rewarding, stating, "I got to do more in two days than I had done in two quarters in the hospital." Each student indicated a significant increase in skill proficiency, communication techniques, problem-solving ability, and self-confidence. Comments such as "I really felt like the nurse" and "Those people really needed me; I saw that I could make a difference" reflect the intangible rewards of such a project.

Agency comments were also very positive. Preceptors noted improvement in the students' nursing skills and confidence levels. Communication skills were evaluated as "significantly improved" during the preceptorship. For example, an agency nurse commented, "The student did all the teaching on Lasix; I did not have anything to add."

EVALUATION OF THE PILOT PROJECT

At the conclusion of this pilot program, three graduates were hired as field nurses in the home health agency. The agency designed a mentorship orientation program, which included a didactic component, as well as field visits with the mentor for a period of 3 to 4 months. Following this experience, the student was given a limited case load, overseen by the mentor. At the conclusion of a 6-month orientation program, the new employee was given a full case load. Agency evaluations reflected the success of this program. Each of the pilot nurses not only has maintained employment within the home health agency but has received internal performance awards and recognition. Both the agency staff and faculty have indicated their intent to continue this program.

REFERENCES

Davies, S., White, E., Riley, E., & Twinn, S. (1996). How can nurse teachers be more effective in practice settings? *Nurse Education Today, 16*(1), 19–27.

Kaiser, K. L., & Rudolph, E. J. (1996). In search of meaning: Identifying competencies relevant to evaluation of the community health nurse generalist. *Journal of Nursing Education, 35*(4), 157–162.

Martin, G. W. (1996). Network: An approach to the facilitation and assessment of critical thinking in nurse education. *Nurse Education Today, 16*(1), 3–9.

Noble, M. A., Redmond, G. M., Williams, J. K., & Langley, C. (1996). Education for the nurse of tomorrow: A community focused curriculum. *Nursing and Health Care: Perspectives on Community, 17*(2), 66–71.

17

Associate Degree Nursing Students Assess Neighborhood Health Care

The Philadelphia Zip Code Project

M. Elaine Tagliareni
Ivory Coleman

Community College of Philadelphia is the only public community college in Philadelphia. The college enrolls approximately 45,000 students; over 70 percent begin courses at the precollege level and over 50 percent are minority. Each year approximately one hundred students graduate from the nursing program. The Department of Nursing has a long tradition of preparing nursing graduates for entry-level positions in acute and long-term care settings. The recent movement to a community-based system of health care necessitated a shift in curriculum focus for the nursing program. The nursing faculty was eager to participate in this national movement and to broaden employment opportunities for graduates in community settings. Like their national community college counterparts, the nursing students at Community College of Philadelphia are intrinsically community based, since they typically live, work, and complete their education within their own community. As graduates, over 90 percent remain in that community and serve their neighbors as nursing professionals.

Faculty realized that, even with their deep commitment to students and to the health of Philadelphians, the nursing department did not know and fully understand the community's health care needs and, sadly, the department and its resources were unknown to the local community. In the spring of 1995, faculty embarked on a project, funded by

210

the Independence Foundation of Philadelphia, to carry out an assessment of the neighborhood adjacent to the college, an area defined by the 19130 zip code. The purpose of the project was threefold: (1) to develop an understanding of the characteristics and health and human service resources in the community; (2) to provide nursing faculty and nursing students with the skill to conduct a community assessment; and (3) to develop linkages with local agencies that provide health promotion and support services to individuals and families across the life span if they reside in the 19130 zip code.

PROJECT DEVELOPMENT

The zip code project evolved over a two-year period and represented a refocusing of initial community initiatives. In the fall of 1994, faculty fully recognized the need to consider student learning experiences in community settings. During the spring semester 1995, four pilot groups of students participated in a two-week clinical placement in a variety of clinical facilities throughout Philadelphia. Clinical experiences included (1) providing intake assessments in the city workers' ambulatory clinic; (2) home health nursing observation visits; (3) screening activities (vision, growth and development, lead poisoning) with Head Start programs; (4) triage activities in a large urban hospital ambulatory medical clinic; and (5) brown bag medicine reviews for older adults with the local Area on Aging. Additionally, some students conducted a preliminary community assessment of the 19130 neighborhood immediately surrounding the college. The notion of "just start" certainly guided activities for that semester.

In developing the pilot project activities, it became apparent that selecting agencies and moving out into Philadelphia, a very large city, was too extensive an undertaking. Faculty needed direction and needed to feel more in control of clinical learning.

With the help of a community health nursing consultant, the pilot project faculty met for a two-day retreat and discussed lessons learned during the community rotations. Faculty developed broad goals for future community experiences and identified a list of assumptions to provide a framework for teaching learning strategies (Figure 17–1). But more importantly, they began to talk about the data collected during the community assessment of the college neighborhood. These discussions revealed

Figure 17–1
Assumptions to Guide Teaching Learning
Decisions in Community Settings

When outcomes guide the clinical learning, faculty can be less prescriptive about how students reach those outcomes.

Every student does not need to have the exact same clinical experiences to meet course and clinical objectives.

Learning in the community does not always work out according to plan and faculty and students need to be flexible about time and agenda.

Students benefit from collegial, colearner relationships with faculty.

With clear outcomes to guide the learning activity, students learn even if the faculty member is not present.

how the assessment had helped faculty understand the social/environmental impact of current health care delivery systems. They had developed a broader outlook toward nursing roles in settings outside acute care and had become aware that many health care services, previously unknown to faculty, existed in the immediate college community. Why not, faculty reasoned, collaborate with agencies "close to home" and meet the nursing needs of the college's neighbors—the residents of the 19130 zip code—rather than attempt to develop relationships with agencies throughout the city? Experiences in the W. K. Kellogg Community College Nursing Home Partnership project had taught faculty the value of building relationships with nursing home residents over an extended period of time to plan nursing care that is personal and comprehensive. Why not apply those same principles to community experiences by returning to the same neighborhood for clinical placements across the curriculum? Reflecting on these questions led faculty to develop the present zip code project. Over the past year, this project has captured the faculty's imagination and interest, provided faculty and students with a vehicle to learn about emerging trends in community-based health care and, most significantly, given faculty and students at every level of the curriculum a common focus for community service initiatives.

PROJECT INTEGRATION

Although the zip code project is, at present, a pilot community experience, learning opportunities outside institutional settings (hospital and nursing home) have been included in the nursing curriculum for a number of years. Faculty incorporated community-based interviews with well-elders, initiated during the Kellogg project (Waters, 1991), into introductory nursing courses, and have developed similar interviews with expectant mothers and with individuals experiencing recent surgical procedures. In later semesters, students follow a family in their local community and study the family's ability to cope and adapt to a family member's long-term chronic health problem. Throughout the nursing program, students plan and implement health fairs, participate in screening programs at Head Start programs and provide intake assessments in ambulatory care settings. Additionally, during first-level nursing courses, students conduct a preliminary assessment of their own neighborhoods (Figure 17–2) in preparation for the more detailed assessment required in the 19130 zip code.

PROJECT GOALS

The zip code project is the capstone experience for community-based learning experiences in the curriculum. This project was conceptualized and designed by faculty to provide students with a beginning understanding of neighborhood health care and to build on the students' previous exposure to community-based health care issues. Faculty anticipated that the activity of collecting data about the college neighborhood would result in an understanding of the health services and nursing needs of the college's neighbors and that, as a result of data collected and relationships initiated during assessment activities, collaborative partnerships would evolve with select community-based agencies. Objectives for the experience (Figure 17–3) were derived through faculty discussions during the retreat and with assistance from Marjorie Buchanan, Community Nurse Consultant and Assistant to the President, Independence Foundation.

Because the nursing faculty at Community College of Philadelphia have been primarily acute care based and share a fundamental orientation to institutional settings, the assessment phase of the project represented a major faculty development initiative. Faculty would become colearners with students, discovering together how families accessed care and how the community functioned as the context for health care delivery. At no time in the planning process did faculty propose that outcomes of the assessment activity would lead to the development of broad community initiatives, a role reserved for the advanced practice nurse.

Figure 17–2
Seminar–N101 Community College of Philadelphia
Department of Nursing

Community Assessment Activity:
Determining Neighborhood Health Care Needs

See Seminar Guide, Week VII for Objectives and Learning Activity Guide.

Describe the community/neighborhood you have chosen to study.

Example: Is it a geographic community (Franklintown or Germantown); is it a community of interest (ethnic, religious, common experience, e.g., AIDS)?

What communities do you belong to?

Neighborhood Assessment Guide (Geographic Community)	Data Collection
A. Type of neighborhood: Residential. Semi-commercial. Urban/metropolitan.	
B. Dwellings in neighborhood: Single-family house. Apartment. Combination.	
C. Age of neighborhood area: Newly constructed. Deteriorating. Foliage (trees, shrubbery).	
D. Sociocultural characteristics: Age composition of residents. Ethnic groups. Employment/unemployment.	
E. Environment: 1. General Safety: Condition of structures, yards, streets, alleys, etc. Traffic patterns. Efficiency of street lighting systems. Availability of fire hydrants. 2. Environmental stressors: Noise. Crime rate. Substance abuse. Crowding. Poverty.	

Figure 17–2 (Continued)

Neighborhood Assessment Guide (Geographic Community)	Data Collection

F. Resources—to what extent are these resources available, if at all?
  Shopping.
  Transportation.
  Recreational.
  Educational.
  Religious.
  Protective services.
  Pharmacies.
  Emergency.
  Human services.
  Newspaper.
 	
G. Neighborhood connection to the health care system:
  What health facilities (hospitals, nursing homes, health dept. clinics, other) are available?
  Where do residents obtain primary health care or other health care?
  What factors contribute to or serve as barriers to using health care facilities?	

What implications can you draw from the data regarding the health care issues for the identified neighborhood?

What are the implications for the nurse when planning discharge for clients from the acute care setting?

Figure 17–3
Community College of Philadelphia
Department of Nursing
The 19130 Project

Purpose: To foster a beginning understanding of the community as the context for health and for health care, in order to prepare nursing students to meet local nursing needs.

Objectives

1. To become familiar with the process and strategies for assessing a community, and factors influencing the health of local families.
2. To develop knowledge and skill in using a collaborative approach to assessment by working with peers, faculty, community representatives, and families in the community.
3. To explore the many factors which affect the health status of families in a community through data collection in a selected neighborhood.
4. To identify how nurses might address nursing needs of families in the selected neighborhood.
5. To discuss the implications for nursing practice in home, community, and institutional settings.
6. To organize and present the information as a contribution to a comprehensive community assessment.

Approach

- Students will be assigned one of the neighborhoods in the 19130 zip code.
- Using a 3-part data collection instrument, students will engage in the following activities during their four day clinical experience with the 19130 Project.

Clinical Day	Data Collection	Post Conference
1	"Walk around" assessment.	What did we see? Whom do we talk with tomorrow?
2	Key informant/resident interviews.	What did we learn? What communication skills were effective?
3	Key informant/resident interviews.	Community perspectives on health and healthcare.
4	Organization of findings.	Group presentation.

DESCRIPTION OF PROJECT
LEARNING ACTIVITIES, SPRING 1996

Community College of Philadelphia's 19130 zip code is a microcosm of Philadelphia with a population that is approximately ⅓ Caucasian, ⅓ African American and ⅓ Hispanic and other minorities. At present, the zip code project student learning experience is 2 to 3 weeks in length and takes place during the fourth semester when students spend a minimum of 5 weeks in the nursing home and 5 to 6 weeks in acute care.

During spring semester 1996, in each 2-week learning experience, 2 of the 12 clinical groups participated. The 2 clinical groups involved approximately 20 clinical students and 2 faculty members. A detailed street map of the 19130 zip code was provided and students were dispatched in groups of three or four to perform a walking assessment of a designated area in the zip code, followed by resident and key informant interviews in that area. For those areas that were furthest away, and on truly inclement weather days, the students drove to their designated area.

Students utilized a Community Assessment Data Collection Instrument developed by faculty and the community consultant to gather information (selected components of the instrument are outlined in Figure 17–4). The data collection instrument is a guideline for information-gathering activities, and students were encouraged to utilize the tool in a variety of ways according to unfolding events and community response. During the pilot experience in spring semester 1996, each student group used different talents and abilities to collect data and to conduct interviews. Some groups spoke primarily to key informants in neighborhood human service agencies, whereas others focused data collection activities on discussions with residents and local merchants. Many of the student groups were racially and culturally mixed so students brought differing perspectives to data collection activities.

On the last of the four clinical days, the groups spent the day on campus compiling information according to guidelines developed by faculty (Figure 17–5). Because the students understood that data collection was a collective activity and that outcomes would build on information gathered by clinical groups, they felt responsible to be accurate and comprehensive. Each student group utilized different approaches to collating data and presenting information. Some developed intricate maps; some focused on one family's approach to health care as a telling example of neighborhood health care access; others discussed ideas to interface

Figure 17–4
The 19130 Project Data Collection Instrument

Areas	Observations and Findings
Part A: Neighborhood Observational Assessment	

Neighborhood Health Care System
1. Health facilities (present/absent)
     Hospitals
     Nursing homes
     Clinics
     Other
2. Sources of primary health care
     District health centers
     Community health centers
     Nursing centers
     Private physicians
     Other

Part B: Key Informants' Perceptions

Health Resources (Available and Absent)
• What health care resources are located in this neighborhood (e.g., people in neighborhood with special expertise, doctors, clinics, hospitals, emergency services, pharmacies)?
• What resources do residents generally use for emergency health care?
• What resources do residents generally use for nonemergency health care?
• Are there resources within the neighborhood for these services, if so, why do people tend to use them or not use them, whichever is the case?

Access/Barriers to Care
• What factors are *most helpful* to residents in their efforts to know about and seek needed health care services?
• What factors *make it difficult* to know about, gain entry into, or use health services?

Part C: Residents' Perceptions

Health and Health Needs
• Is health a major concern in your household, or are there other things facing you that are more urgent?
• What does "being healthy" mean to you and your family?
• What kinds of things do you and your family do in order to be healthy?

Figure 17–4 (Continued)

Areas	Observations and Findings
Health and Health Needs cont'd • What are the most common health needs facing your family and perhaps other families in the neighborhood? • Are there health problems in the neighborhood that affect many families and are becoming an issue of community concern? *Health Resources* • What health resources do your family use most frequently? • Where does your family go for emergency health care? • Where does your family go for such health care services as pregnancy care, checkups for babies and children, checkups for adults, treatment for periodic illnesses, etc.? *Paying for Health Care* • How do most families in this neighborhood pay for their health care services (pay in cash, Medicaid enrollment, managed care plan, private insurance)? • If families are unable to pay, where do they go for health care? *Access/Barriers to Care* • In scheduling appointments, what do you find is helpful and what is difficult in this process? • Once you have an appointment for services, are there things that make it difficult to keep the appointment (in your home, the community and the health care setting)? • When you arrive for your appointment, how do you find the experience: from point of registration, waiting, seeing your provider, scheduling follow-up care, or other factors? • Do you have any recommendations about things that would make learning about health care services, making appointments, for how services are provided, or any other factors that would make health care easier to obtain for you, your family, and perhaps other neighborhood families?	

Figure 17–5
Community College of Philadelphia Department of Nursing
The 19130 Project Guidelines for
Summary Presentation of Findings

I. Introduction
  - Members of group.
  - Name of neighborhood.
  - Geographic boundaries for data collection activities.

II. Approach to Data Collection
  - *Neighborhood walk around* (How you proceeded; degree of difficulty in getting around; feelings as you moved about, etc.)
  - *Key informants/residents* (How were they identified; who were they; how did they feel about participating; was the information they provided reflective of commonly held or differing perspectives?)

III. Description of Neighborhood and the Residents
  - What was the general appearance of the neighborhood?
  - Who are the people who live here?
  - What are the lifeways of the community?
  - What are the overall strengths and limitations of the neighborhood?

IV. Description of Residents' Health
  - What are the residents' definitions of health and general approach to health care?
  - What health needs, problems, issues, and concerns were identified or raised by residents?
  - How do residents typically use health care services?
  - What health resources are present and which are absent in the neighborhood?
  - How do residents pay for health care services?
  - How accessible are health care services generally?
  - What factors serve as barriers to care for residents?

V. Conclusions and Recommendations

Summarized data collection instrument to be submitted by each clinical group.

neighborhood agencies that were unaware of similar agencies in the immediate community.

The issue of student safety was of paramount importance to faculty throughout the zip code project. Students were instructed to remain in their groups of three or four and to remove themselves from any situation that did not "feel right." No incidents placing students in jeopardy occurred during the semester. But it was the number one concern described by students in their weekly logs:

Approaching people I didn't know frightened me. Yet the experience of interacting with the public in a personal and yet professional way was the most rewarding part of the assessment.

I was initially concerned about safety, about not knowing what was really expected of us and whether people would want to talk with us. But talking to people about health care and about their experiences will make me a more conscientious nurse.

EDUCATIONAL OUTCOMES

Increase in Cultural Sensitivity

The dialogue in postconferences throughout the project was always lively and intense. Faculty were struck by the students' honesty and forthright analysis of culturally sensitive issues. Some students, for the first time, interacted as a nurse in environments where their cultural group was dominant. These students spoke frankly about what it meant to them to be accepted and recognized as a professional among their own cultural group and how difficult it had been for them to practice in the hospital, where "white ways" are the decision-making framework. For other students, this was the first time that they had considered health care to be culturally based. Throughout the program of learning at Community College of Philadelphia, students participate in cultural sensitivity seminars, but for many students, this was the first time that they had experienced the issue in practice. Many eyes and hearts were opened during those postconference discussions.

Ability to Cope with Ambiguity

The community assessment activity seemed unstructured to students accustomed to the rituals of clinical experience in institutional settings. Although students had the data collection tool as a guide, the initial walk-around assessment (Figure 17–4, Part A) elicited comments in the preconference discussions:

- "What is expected of me? How will I be perceived by the community?"
- "Finding out exactly what we should be doing is my first concern. It is very unclear to me."

Students challenged faculty to give them "the answers" and to tell them how to collect essential data. Faculty listened to their initial concerns and encouraged them to problem-solve with their small groups to plan approaches collaboratively and then to "just start." Each time a new clinical group joined the project, faculty felt the transfer of their anxiety, and each time faculty were surprised, once again, to hear students in the final postconference comment that one of the primary benefits of the experience was the confidence they now had in their ability to complete data collection. Students were proud of their ability to work through initial uncertainty and to discover information previously unknown to their peers and to the faculty. Self-confidence, a characteristic of critical thinkers, was a striking outcome of the students' activities and reflected a willingness by faculty to allow for a less prescribed clinical experience.

Enhancement of Critical Thinking

Over the past several years, faculty have defined critical thinking skills to include discovery learning, challenging of assumptions, reflection, and understanding of context. Faculty discovered that the zip code project, as a teaching strategy, facilitated development of these essential components. Working in groups, students participated in discovery learning and focused inquiry and challenged assumptions about how individuals and families accessed health care in the community and how and why families made decisions about utilization of neighborhood resources. Students were encouraged by faculty to reflect on their experiences in order to change their perspective on health care delivery patterns.

> *I was totally enlightened to the many factors that determine one's health status and attitude. I didn't realize all the barriers which existed in one's attempt to seek access to health care.*
> *I am much more aware of the many barriers faced by countless people regarding health care. I now have a new perception regarding people who seek health care in the 19130 community.*

Opportunity to Reframe Thinking about Current Nursing Practice

Students reported that experiences in the zip code helped them to understand the full spectrum of health care and to appreciate the hospital as a transitional setting.

Seeing how health care is provided, not just in a structured setting such as a hospital, but in people's communities, helped me understand holistic care for the first time.

FUTURE PLANS

After just one semester of assessment activities, the nursing department has become known in the 19130 community. Already the nursing department has been asked to participate in community health fairs and other outreach activities. At present, the department has established collaborative relationships with zip code agencies, such as a Head Start program, an elementary school, a church-affiliated homebound elderly program, a 200-unit high-rise senior citizen housing complex, an AIDS hospice, and an ambulatory care clinic.

Although the faculty's initial intent was to consider the 19130 community assessment only as a mechanism to learn about the local community, the activity itself proved to be so valuable that future fourth-semester students will continue to use the data collection tool to assess the neighborhood. Discovery learning, in the context of a collaborative teaching learning environment may be the most significant outcome of zip code activities. Faculty plan to combine the assessment and service components of the zip code project during the second year of project implementation. The zip code project now represents, both for faculty and students, the nursing department's response and commitment to an emerging, community-based health care system. In his weekly log, a nursing student tellingly wrote:

Being involved in a project that needed doing for years, reinforced for me, the "community" that is part of Community College of Philadelphia's name. What took so long?

REFERENCES

Waters, V. (Ed.). (1991). *Teaching gerontology.* New York: National League for Nursing Press.

18

A Community of Their Own

Clinical Experiences in Subsidized Housing Sites

Jean Haspeslagh

Providing nursing students with experiences that allow them to learn and internalize the concepts of community health nursing while also developing self-confidence and independence is a challenge community health nursing faculty face with each new class. Finding clinical sites where students not only will care for individuals in the community but also will deal with meeting the needs of aggregates within the community is an ongoing concern, especially for faculty teaching in schools that are not located in large urban areas. This need for community-focused experiences becomes more and more important as schools of nursing strive to prepare their graduates to function in a health care system that is turning to community-based care as one answer to cost containment.

In the past, students' community health experiences have included observational or limited participation in health department clinics and assorted community-based agencies (e.g., mental health centers, student health services, after-hours clinics), assignments "riding" with the home health nurse, and home visits to selected clients (individuals and/or families). Students who made visits with a nurse had opportunities to observe the community health nurse in action but often failed to identify with the key elements associated with that role.

To make the role of the community health nurse more real for students, some schools provided students with the opportunity to make "solo" visits to individuals or families in the community. These experiences were not without their own problems:

1. Finding adequate and appropriate numbers of individuals or families for students to visit.

2. Finding assigned persons at home. As all community health nurses know, frequently families on health department rosters (a) don't have phones, (b) relocate without notice, (c) don't answer the phone, (d) don't respond to someone at the door, or (e) even if contacted and agreeing to the visit aren't there when the student attempts to visit—Why? They forgot, were at the store, went out to lunch, or just "got a better offer."

3. Students' motivation can also be a problem. Occasionally, the instructor has to wonder: Did the student really try? Was the family really gone that many times? What was really going on? Did the student conveniently not find the family because of feeling uncomfortable with home visits, with working with persons from different cultural or ethnic groups, with persons in lower socioeconomic neighborhoods?

4. Supervision of student visits presents difficulties especially if the family/patient does not have a telephone. Logistics (number of students, time constraints, and distances) limit the number of visits the faculty member can make with each student.

5. Lastly, seeing the broader picture of community is often difficult for students who are accustomed to dealing with individuals with the emphasis on their medical diagnoses. When assigned to an individual in the community, they still tend to focus on the individual's medical conditions—even when they are seeing a family.

ONE PROGRAM'S EXPERIENCE

In an attempt to address the preceding problems, community health nursing clinical experiences were sought that provided baccalaureate nursing students with the opportunity to apply community health concepts with groups of clients. It was important that the experience allowed students to work with individuals, families, and groups and provided the opportunity to address health promotion, health maintenance, and health education issues. An ongoing part of the curriculum was related to incorporation of clients' cultural beliefs into the plan of care and for community health this became a major objective. In addition, a community assessment project was to be conducted by each clinical group. This project included not only the assessment but the development of a plan of action and the implementation of that plan with the population assessed. This project was in addition to the weekly clinical laboratory experiences.

Selection of a Community

While serving as a member of a Family/Neighborhood Task Force through the local DREAM (Drug-Free Resources for Education and Alternatives in Mississippi) program, the needs of various neighborhoods represented on this committee became evident. It also became clear that nursing students could be ideal persons to provide assistance and intervention in these neighborhoods especially in the areas of health maintenance, health promotion, and health education activities. The apartment managers of three apartment complexes expressed an interest and were eager to have nursing students involved in their neighborhoods.

The first site selected was a three-story apartment building with subsidized housing specifically designated for elderly and handicapped individuals. This site consisted of 50 apartments with 54 residents, primarily of an older ethnically mixed group ranging in age from 54 to 93. There also were a few younger persons with physical disabilities including visual impairments and paraplegia. The second site comprised 12 buildings with a total of 90 apartments. Residents again presented an ethnically mixed group. It included single young adults, married young adults, young families, single-parent families, and elders. Persons living at this site included those with chronic illness, pregnant women, and newborns.

Arrangements were made with the managers and a letter of agreement was signed by the director of the school of nursing and the apartment manager. This letter clearly stated that the focus of the students' experience would be on health assessment, health promotion, and health education activities. It was emphasized that residents were free to participate or not as they desired.

The sites chosen notified residents that nursing students would be coming to work with them. This was done in three ways: apartment newsletters, letters/flyers sent to residents and posted on bulletin boards, and announcements at residents' meetings. Space—usually a group meeting room—was provided for students and faculty to gather and to use as a home base. This allowed the faculty member to be on site but still permitted student autonomy when interacting with the residents. Thus the faculty member was able to serve as consultant and troubleshooter for the student. Students were encouraged to problem-solve and discuss possible solutions with their group and then bring the proposed solutions to the faculty member.

What resulted was that the sites provided students with minicommunities. To reduce student anxiety and to facilitate accomplishment of one of the course objectives related to working in groups, students were placed in work groups of two to four persons. In the three-story apartment building, three or four students were assigned to each floor, while students at the multibuilding complex were assigned in pairs to two or three buildings.

Preparation for the Experience

To prepare the students for this clinical experience, faculty set aside time during the orientation to the course and again during the orientation to clinical for discussion of students' expectation and concerns about their pending clinical laboratory experiences. Students were asked to identify barriers they anticipated and how they would address those barriers. The discussion, with peer input and group problem-solving, decreased anxiety about the unexpected and provided an opportunity to address the myths and stereotypes attributed to the neighborhoods where the students were assigned. Safety issues were also discussed at this time.

During the clinical orientation, the apartment managers and a former Vista volunteer who worked in and lives in the multibuilding project met with the students before they began working with the residents. They provided overviews of the respective sites and the residents living there. They openly discussed the probability that initially residents might seem hesitant to open up and share but that hesitancy would diminish once trust was established. They reminded students that oftentimes residents are hesitant because they fear that some agency may want to take something away from them or cause trouble. Students were encouraged to express their fears and doubts, and the managers and the Vista volunteer honestly responded to those concerns. Taking time for this dialogue was critical for the success of the experience.

Potential Barriers Identified by the Students

Potential barriers most frequently identified by students were primarily related to themselves, not to the site. Lack of self-confidence and uncertainty about own abilities were at the top of the list, followed by concerns regarding being more autonomous. Students also felt that communication barriers might be a problem. Students were honest in their self-assessment and felt that being nonjudgmental was a potential barrier. Ineffective time management and poor preparation for clinical were identified as additional handicaps to a successful experience. Barriers identified that related to the neighborhoods and the sites were primarily fear of the unknown and expectations that the environment would be unclean.

Students' expectations of the experience reflected all the stereotypes attributed to lower socioeconomic neighborhoods and subsidized housing. Students anticipated unclean rundown apartments, vastly different values, and a totally unsafe environment. Students discovered that, for the most part, residents held the same or similar values as the students, lived in clean homes in which they took pride, and were more receptive to the students than they expected. As one student described it: "The homes were much like my own and those of my friends, some were spotless, some cluttered, and some dirty." Another explained: "My fears have decreased greatly. I have come to realize this is home for my clients and is an important place to them just as my home is to me."

Clinical Requirements

Students in the community health course were expected to accomplish a number of things while in this course. A key element that assists the faculty member in determining whether students met course objectives was the use of a clinical log or journal with student goals for the overall experience, weekly goals, and personal reflections. Self-evaluation was expected each week and at the end of the experience. The log provided a mechanism for students to record their assessments, their plans, and their interventions, as well as to evaluate the successfulness of those interventions. Students were expected to record their own assessment of their community in their log. They also used the log to reflect on the events of the day, their perceptions, and their feelings about the experiences. The faculty, in turn, could dialogue with the students through notations and responses to students' reflections. This log was not graded but was required for successful completion of the clinical experience.

Semester goals set by the students contained a common core:

- Improving time management skills.
- Improving assessment skills.
- Improving interpersonal/communication skills.
- Increasing the awareness of the roles of the community health nurse.
- Increasing knowledge of community resources.
- Developing more autonomy.
- Recognizing own prejudices and attempting to develop sensitivity.

Students having their clinical experiences in these settings were expected to assess residents who were willing to participate in the project. They were also expected to determine both individual and community (their floor or apartment buildings) health promotion, health maintenance, and health education needs. Once needs were identified, the students then described how those needs could best be met through interventions: one to one, in a family, or in a group setting. The student work groups were expected to consider the needs of multiple residents (e.g., diabetes, arthritis, hypertension, cardiac problems) and address them. Medication-related issues were also addressed. Students then developed a plan of care that included the most appropriate interventions. This plan was then implemented either with the individual, the family, or with groups of residents.

The most common needs identified in the single building apartment for the elderly and handicapped fell into two categories: physical conditions and psychosocial/economic. The most common physical problems of the residents were hypertension, diabetes, cardiovascular-related problems, and paraplegia. Dietary problems and exercise/activity-related issues affecting or affected by the physical conditions were also addressed. The psychosocial/economic problems most frequently identified included depression, chronic mental illness, family/relationship issues, isolation, and problems associated with limited income.

The needs identified by the students working at the multibuilding complex were slightly different. Again, they fell into two categories:

physical and psychosocial/economic. The most frequently identified physical problems were related to hypertension, diabetes, pregnancy, child health, diet, and medications. Psychosocial/economic needs for this population were related to stress, parenting, school truancy, and a major area—self-concept.

Students' interventions with the residents were as varied as the populations that made up the communities. Interventions that were delivered on a one-to-one basis frequently consisted of teaching, especially regarding specific medications or treatments a resident was using. In one instance, a resident was having problems assembling a new inhaler and the directions were unclear. The student called the pharmacist, received instructions, and then taught the client the proper method. Instructions regarding special diets and medication were frequent. Working with residents with elevated blood pressures or blood sugars often involved encouraging them to contact their physician.

Interventions with families, again, focused on teaching. Areas taught included such things as normal growth and development and realistic expectations of children based on their age, emotional support for persons caring for an ill spouse or family member, dealing with an alcoholic or addicted family member, and parenting skills. Students worked with a single mother of triplets and with an elderly grandmother who cared for her grandchildren. One student assisted a resident with her attempts at setting limits on her adult children who often took advantage of her.

Community-focused interventions were varied and ranged from teaching to activities. Group teaching for common health problems such as hypertension and diabetes were frequently conducted. Chair exercise classes were well received by the older population. After identifying that children at the multibuilding complex had bicycles that were in disrepair, students conducted a bicycle clinic where they adjusted and tightened seats and handlebars and inflated tires. This provided an ideal time for talking with the children about safety, staying in school and other concerns. A session on identifying common childhood illnesses and recognizing when to take the child to the doctor or emergency room was made available to parents and grandparents.

Students' Evaluations of the Experience

Students' evaluations of their experiences in these community health clinical sites reflected successful achievement of their goals, particularly those goals associated with the roles of the community health nurse, communications/interpersonal relationships skills, assessment skills, community resources, autonomy, and increased cultural sensitivity. As one student expressed, "I accomplished more than I realized." A second reported, "We were in an atmosphere that promoted autonomy." Another reflected, "It was an experience that gave opportunities to make it okay or great. It was up to us."

Reflecting back on the anticipated barriers, most students were amazed to find residents so appreciative of what they were doing. A social worker living and working in the neighborhood surrounding one of the apartments related how the residents living there found that the presence of the nursing students and the faculty member gave them an increased sense of worth; someone cared enough to come into their neighborhood. Students found people began to wave at them when they entered the neighborhood. Residents at both complexes made a concerted effort to let the faculty member know how important the students' presence was for them and for their neighborhood. Students found this affirmation increased their own self-confidence and sense of well-being.

A Faculty Member's Perspective

From the faculty perspective, having the community health experience in subsidized housing sites demonstrated the realities of community health nursing to students and simplified their supervision. The faculty member on site provided students with easy access to consultation, yet still allowed students to experience independence. It also made it possible for the faculty member to serve as a role model through interactions with residents and staff in the apartments. Students began to seek out the faculty members' opinions and ideas without feeling that they would be criticized if they did not have all the answers. At the same time, faculty became aware of some of the students' creative ways to address the health needs of their communities.

IN THEIR OWN WORDS

The reactions to having a community health experience in the neighborhoods of subsidized housing projects can best be summarized in the students' own words. With their permission, the students in N427 Community Health Nursing Practicum speak:

I spent an hour with a man, just talking. After leaving, I felt like I had helped him with nothing. I got thinking, and I realized that wasn't true. I had listened.

Another student reflected:

This week, I learned the difference between "Supernurse" and a super nurse. "Supernurse" feels the need to be inhuman and try to fix all what ails. A super nurse is human and not afraid to admit that and that he or she might not know all the answers. But, what they do is take the time to find them.

The experience of working with residents from different cultural and ethnic backgrounds evoked the following reflection:

The more time I spent working with these clients, the more I realized that they are just like me. They have the same worries and concerns . . . as I do . . . I don't share some of the same problems but they have the same basic needs as I:

> *Someone to talk to*
> *Hoping to better themselves*
> *Worries about making some kind of*
> *   difference no matter how*
> *   trivial it may seem to others*
> *Health concerns*
> *Money concerns.*

In conclusion, I borrow the words of yet another student:

We not only taught and talked—We listened and learned.

19

The Alliance for Health Model

Helping Students to Understand Community Health Assessment and Care Delivery

Stephen Paul Holzemer

The Alliance for Health Model provides a blueprint to help students understand community health assessment and care delivery. One concern with contemporary nursing education is that some graduates find it difficult to adjust to the expectations of the workforce in community-based settings. The Alliance for Health Model (Holzemer & Arnold, in press) should assist nurses and students in making the transition to practitioner because it offers a view of health and illness that is (1) reflected in the contemporary literature (Hicks, Stallmeyer, & Coleman, 1993; Shugars, O'Neil, & Bader, 1991); (2) open to validation by practitioners and educators on an ongoing basis, and (3) can be used in continuing education programs in hospitals, community-based settings, and formal education settings in schools of nursing.

This presentation of the model defines the components of the model and identifies some of the ways the model can be used in nursing education settings. The term student refers to both the generic student in a nursing program and nurses who are receiving retraining for community-based care. The core ideas about the Alliance Model originated from a work group of care providers and educators mapping out the needed mind and body skills for community-based practice. The components of the model and examples of how it is used in education activities are included in this discussion.

COMPONENTS OF THE MODEL

The five components of the model include an examination of:

1. Community-based needs.
2. Care management techniques.
3. Influences on resource allocation decisions.

The context for how community-based needs, care management techniques, and influences on resource allocation decisions relate to each other is a combination of:

4. The expertise of the interdisciplinary team.
5. Validation of services by the client.

Figure 19–1 provides a visual representation of the model.

Using the Alliance for Health Model allows students to view health concerns beyond a narrow nursing perspective. It encourages students and hospital-based nurses to view health problems from a community perspective. Each of the five components of the model is considered essential to working in the community and making proper nursing judgments about the care that nurses need to provide. Nurses have a role in assessing each of the five essential components.

Community-Based Needs

Community-based needs include but are not restricted to the assessment and analysis of the following sources of information:

1. Patterns of morbidity and mortality.
2. Demographics (age, gender, education level, income, housing).
3. Environmental concerns.
4. Public services (fire, police, sanitation, education, recreation, and sports).
5. Aesthetics (art, music, culture, religion).
6. Health-related facilities (hospitals, community-based organizations [CBOs], subacute and custodial care facilities, public health facilities, home care organizations).

Figure 19–1
The Alliance for Health Model for Community Health
Assessment and Care Delivery

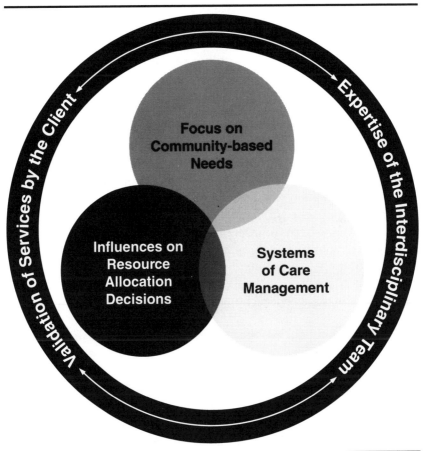

The way community-based needs are met or not met is a reflection of how professionals and the public manage care and allocate resources. Since each community has unique health care needs, nurses and others need to continuously reevaluate their use of the nursing process to accurately assess community needs.

Care Management Techniques

The management of health care is a complex phenomenon and includes the mix of client problems, the expectations of the public for care, the competence of professionals, the accepted standards of care, and the use of interdisciplinary care plans or action plans. Care management techniques develop and change according to the evolution of health care problems (community-based needs) and decisions about how populations allocate resources.

Influences on Resource Allocation Decisions

A number of variables influence how resource allocation decisions are made. They include patterns of resource allocation; the values and beliefs of the population; the reliance on local, regional, and federal government funding; the influence of special interest groups on resource allocation; and patterns of insurance coverage.

In any community, one or more of these variables may influence resource allocation decisions at the same time. The major influences on how health care resources are allocated are associated with the skill evident in care management techniques and the volume and complexity of community-based needs.

Expertise of the Interdisciplinary Team

The expertise of the interdisciplinary team depends on the involvement of all disciplines giving care. Although each team member will be somewhere on the continuum between expert and novice, the team as a whole needs to be competent to care for the public's health (Tresolini & the Pew-Fetzer Task Force, 1994). With varied expertise, the team will necessarily have the resources to make necessary referrals within the group and outside the group. Team members need to work together successfully to make a positive difference in the care people receive (Holzemer, 1995; National League for Nursing, 1993).

Validation of Services by the Client

Health care services need to be available, accessible, affordable, appropriate, adequate, and acceptable (Krout, 1994). Only the client can validate health-related services that are important from his or her perspective. Certain vulnerable populations such as prisoners, children, and people with severe neurological function will need to have others act for them to validate services. If it is impossible to validate services with the client or the client's agent, as with a health care proxy, the provider should offer services that reflect a general standard of care. Standards of care are generated by professionals who are charged with defining safe and prudent care.

LEARNING ACTIVITIES

Community-Based Needs, Care Management Techniques and Influences on Resource Allocation Decisions

Table 19–1 lists some of the questions that can be given to students to expand their understanding of the community. These learning activities assist them to use the first three components of the Alliance Model for Health. After experience with the model, students create their own questions to assess client needs. Students begin the process of assessing communities by sharpening their critical thinking skills. Creative questions for community assessment can be directed to geographic, political, and special interest as well as ethnic communities.

Expertise of the Interdisciplinary Team

To assist learners to appreciate the expertise of the interdisciplinary team, the learner can ask care providers to solve problems from their professional perspective. Learners can compare how providers make referrals and turn to others for assistance. An example follows.

Kerly Ramon Needs Home Care

> Ms. Kerly Ramon is scheduled for discharge and makes last-minute plans to recover at a relative's home in another state. Ms. Ramon has transient ischemic attacks and has trouble remembering to take her four prescription drugs. Ms. Ramon mentions that her bedroom will be on the second floor of her relative's home.

Study questions include: What are the differences in how nurses, social workers, physicians, or others solve potential problems? What resources are available in a 50–100 mile radius to provide support to lay caregivers?

Table 19–1
Learning Activities Using the Alliance Model for Health

Learning Activity	Community-Based Needs	Care Management Techniques	Resource Allocation
Students visit a HIV/AIDS day care center to better understand the needs of this population.	How are clients cared for with neurological and motor function deficits?	Describe the process for establishing day care services? How is day care for people living with HIV different from elder care?	How is the day care center funded? How did the neighborhood respond to the establishment of the day care program?
Phone calls are made to people who visited the emergency department for nonemergent problems.	Describe the types of problems seen in the emergency department. Ask the clients why they use the emergency department for care.	Explain how non-emergent problems are handled in the department. How accurate is the client's recall of instructions and teaching?	Compare the cost of a clinic visit with an emergency department visit.
Clinics for high-risk pregnancy are attended to provide care to people of different backgrounds and learn about childcare from different cultural perspectives.	Compare the pregnancy rates and premature birth rates with those of other communities. Into what types of family units are children born?	What is the make up of health professionals working in different parts of the city/town? How do care providers approach the care of clients from different cultures?	What are the sources of funding for high-risk pregnancy?
Students visit a soup kitchen to observe group process among the homeless population.	What are the demographics of this population? What are the security concerns of the staff when working with this population? Are these concerns founded?	How are health-related problems addressed in this group? Are the staff trained in CPR or the Heimlich maneuver?	Who advocates for the needs of the homeless? What is the pattern of soup kitchen services for the community? Are these services offered seven days a week and year round?

Students learn about other professions by interviewing other care providers for how they solve problems important to their clients. Students can begin to understand the process of referral and delegation as it relates to the work of the interdisciplinary team.

Validation of Services by the Client

To appreciate the meaning of validation of services for clients, students as future users (clients) of the care system can prioritize and discuss services they consider to be essential. Students can negotiate for the

Table 19–2
Creating Services for a Community

Healthcareville is a small town 150 miles from the nearest major city. The community has decided to begin a clinic and needs to decide which services to provide. From the list provided, identify the five services that you think are necessary for the health of the town. The following statistics reflect the population of Healthcareville (blank spaces can be used to vary the health care needs).

a. Average age of residents _____ .
b. 42% Black/Latino (a).
c. Leading causes of death (1) _____ , (2) _____ , (3) _____ .
d. 34% Single Parents.
e. Other variables _____ .

Choose 5 services that you think are essential for this community. Work in groups to negotiate a final list of services.

_____ Hospice beds for respite
_____ 4 intensive care beds
_____ MRI scanner
_____ 10 skilled nursing beds
_____ 3 home care nurses
_____ Meals on Wheels services
_____ Breast cancer center
_____ 10 hrs/week midwife
_____ Sports medicine physical therapist
_____ Adolescent antiviolence program
_____ Orthopedic medical services
_____ Emergicenter

services that are important to them while appreciating that there is a wide range of services that clients (or other students) may want.

The exercise illustrated in Table 19–2 assists students with setting their own priorities as well as negotiating with others in the allocation of resources that are important to them.

The demographics of Healthcareville can be changed so students learn how the needs of people may differ because of the characteristics of the population. Additional exercises related to resource allocation can be created by further limiting the services available in the community, or by suggesting additional services.

SUMMARY

The five components of the Alliance for Health Model are:

1. Community-based needs.
2. Care management techniques.
3. Influences on resource allocation decisions.
4. The expertise of the interdisciplinary team.
5. Validation of services by the client.

The Alliance for Health Model can be used to teach both students and nurses in practice about community-based care. Learners who obtain a larger appreciation for community-based care should be able to view acute care hospital-based nursing from a more realistic perspective. Increased skill in community assessment is a marketable trait nurses need to refine as they reengineer their skills and knowledge base for future practice.

REFERENCES

Hicks, L. L., Stallmeyer, J. M., & Coleman, J. R. (1993). *Role of the nurse in managed care*. Washington, DC: American Nurses Publishing.

Holzemer, S. P. (1995). Council of Community Health Services (CCHS) confronts issues in community-based and managed care. *NLN Update, 1*(1), 5.

Holzemer, S. P., & Arnold, J. (in press). Alliance for health: A model for community health assessment. In M. Klainberg, S. P. Holzemer, M. Leonard, J. Arnold, & T. M. Graf (Eds.), *Community health nursing*. New York: McGraw-Hill.

Krout, J. A. (Ed.). (1994). *Providing community-based services to the rural elderly.* Thousand Oakes, CA: Sage.

National League for Nursing. (1993). *A vision for nursing education.* New York: Author.

Shugars, D. A., O'Neil, E. H., & Bader, J. D. (1991). *Healthy America: Practitioners for 2005, an agenda for action for U. S. health professional schools.* Durham, NC: Pew Health Professions Commission.

Tresolini, C. P., & the Pew-Fetzer Task Force. (1994). *Health Professions Education and relationship-centered care.* San Francisco: Pew Health Professions Commission.

20

A Community Nursing Center Provides Health Care for the Homeless

Joan Wilk
Vicky Talbert

People who are homeless, the uninsured, and the underinsured continue to have difficulty finding health care services that are accessible and affordable. According to some estimates, the homeless with mental illness make up one-third of the homeless population and experience this difficulty to an even greater degree due to their social isolation and the stigma associated with mental illness (U.S. Department of Health and Human Services, 1992). As health care costs soar and resources dwindle, a rising political tide favors provision of health care for those who are publicly or privately insured. The homeless, with transient life styles and geographic instability, seldom fall into either category.

The heightened concern about funds for Medicare, reform for Medicaid, rising insurance rates, and paying the growing medical bills of municipal, county, state, and federal employees has eclipsed the plight of the uninsured and underinsured. Entitlement to health care seems to frame the debate in the United States and it is a debate in which the homeless are not included. Nevertheless, the number of people who are homeless continues to grow and their need for health care continues to be a harsh reality.

LITERATURE REVIEW

Characteristics of the Homeless

The changing demographics of homelessness, particularly family homelessness, are proof that anyone can become homeless. Women and children are believed to make up one-third of the homeless with single women comprising approximately 12 percent of the homeless population (Francis, 1992). While the average age of the homeless person is believed to be around 35 years, it is estimated that 14.8 to 28 percent of the homeless are age 50 and older (Elias & Inui, 1993). As many as one out of every three homeless people may suffer from a major mental illness such as schizophrenia or depression (U.S. Department of Health and Human Services, 1992). Although estimates vary and census figures for the homeless have been criticized for methodological flaws, it is believed that annually one to two million people are homeless (Blau, 1992).

Health Care for the Homeless

Rising health care costs affect everyone. The homeless, however, are particularly hard-hit since they are among the growing numbers of the uninsured. The lack of funds for community alternatives, even more than deinstitutionalization, has compounded the problem for the mentally ill. Without resources, they account for a disproportionate percentage of the homeless in need of health care. They experience a variety of health problems. Hypertension and cardiac problems, respiratory infections and disease, dermatological conditions, and social isolation are among the prevalent health care problems of the homeless (Hodnicki, 1990). These conditions have a tendency to become chronic due to the real and perceived barriers to health care. Of particular concern is the perception by the homeless of the negative behaviors of health care providers that discourage the seeking of care (Ursatine, Gelberg, Smith, & Lesser, 1994).

THE NEED FOR HEALTH PROMOTION AND ILLNESS PREVENTION

Nurses encounter the homeless in varied health care settings. Hospitals, health departments, and community clinics are some of the sites where health care for the homeless is delivered. Opportunities for situational health promotion and intervention can arise in hallways and waiting rooms just as they do at soup kitchens and shelters. They may occur during planned visits or when clients are seeking help for acute problems.

Because of the episodic use of health care services by the homeless, nurses who work in acute care and community settings are often at a loss for helpful strategies when their clients are homeless. The health care needs of the homeless are complex. They lack insurance, access to health care, and social support, and are often unable to engage in activities that will increase their level of wellness. They may miss appointments due to their highly mobile lifestyle, or the lack of transportation, or because food and shelter needs seem more urgent to them. These factors often prevent the homeless client from seeking care until an acute situation has developed. Treatment may be sought as a last resort for a condition that would have been amenable to earlier intervention.

The attitudes and behaviors of the nurse are particularly important as they influence the homeless person's decision to use limited health resources wisely and earlier. Seeking early treatment and solving problems before they are exacerbated is the first step toward health promotion. To promote health successfully, the nurse must understand the needs, culture, and life situation of persons and families who are homeless. With this understanding as a basis, nurses will find it easier to deliver health care in a nonjudgmental, respectful, and relevant manner.

There are similarities in the health promotion interventions for the homeless and the general population. Certain lifestyle behaviors that interfere with the achievement of optimum wellness, such as smoking, poor nutrition, inadequate exercise, stress and misuse of alcohol and drugs, are shared by members of each group. However, many homeless people have critical, often unique, needs that must be considered in the context of their long periods of homelessness when addressing those health issues. This includes prevention of homelessness-related illnesses, managing the challenges of shelter or street living, maintaining personal hygiene, and negotiating health care and other institutional systems. Low self-esteem, ineffective coping skills, lack of parenting knowledge, inadequate interpersonal skills and poor social support may increase the risk that clients with mental illness will remain homeless or be candidates for repeated episodes of homelessness (Berne, Dato, Mason, & Rafferty, 1990). Interventions in these areas by health providers can reduce this risk.

A NURSING CENTER RESPONDS
TO HOMELESS CLIENTS

In many communities, homelessness presents a particular challenge due to the lack of local resources and, in some cases, a reluctance to acknowledge a community problem that is not always apparent. For every homeless person who is visible on the streets, in the parks, and in public buildings and shelters, there are many others who are the "hidden" homeless. They are the people who find shelter with friends, in single room occupancy apartments, or in shabby motels. Some of them live in cars, garages, or under bridges. Many go relatively unnoticed by other members of their communities until they seek help from local shelters and soup kitchens.

It was in this setting, at an emergency shelter and soup kitchen site in a small Midwestern city, that a group of nurses and nursing students established a Community Nursing Center to work with homeless "guests." The guests are people who have an evening meal at the soup kitchen and those who are temporarily sheltered at the same site. The operational definition of homelessness used in this setting is that of the Stewart B. McKinney Homeless Assistance Act of 1987: Homeless people are those who lack a fixed, regular, and adequate nighttime residence. Since the service began in 1992, the nurses have provided health promotion, education, and primary health care during approximately 1,400 visits from the homeless each year.

The people who seek services are those without health care due to a lack of "connectedness" with the social welfare system, low-paying jobs without insurance, or the inability to access primary health care when and where it is needed. The on-site professionally staffed Community Nursing Center has become the entry point into the health care system for many of the homeless in the community.

The establishment of the Community Nursing Center was a logical response to the lack of access to care. It provides homeless persons and families direct access to health promotion, illness prevention, and illness management services in a community-based setting that this population has already identified as accessible. A nurse practitioner, a BSN prepared community health nurse, and an MSN nurse whose specialty is community mental health collaborate on client health issues and case management to provide care that promotes optimum health among the clients.

Primarily supported by a grant from the Division of Nursing, Department of Health and Human Services, health care is provided to clients without charge. The Community Nursing Center offers a variety of educational experiences for nursing students. Each year, the nurses are role models and teachers to approximately 40 baccalaureate nursing students at all educational levels who spend clinical time at the Nursing Center.

Annually, a senior preceptor student and eight sophomore students spend an entire semester participating in Community Nursing Center activities.

STRATEGIES FOR INTERVENTION
WITH HOMELESS CLIENTS

To provide guidelines for working with the homeless, nurses at the Community Nursing Center identified a number of strategies for intervention aimed at fostering a nurse-client relationship where health promotion and illness prevention can occur. Although the strategies were developed for use in a homeless shelter, they would be appropriate in any community-based setting or in acute care settings. The strategies form the foundation for health promotion interventions that assist homeless individuals and families in maintaining and improving health, preventing injury and disease, and developing healthier lifestyle behaviors.

Create a Client-Friendly Environment   Providing warm, comfortable surroundings and greeting the clients by name demonstrate respect and encourage them to engage in dialogue about health promotion and lifestyle changes. When clients were asked to evaluate the health care they received at the Community Nursing Center, they related their satisfaction with nursing care to the importance of having the nurses call them by name, welcome them to the Community Nursing Center, and indicate a willingness to help. Walk-in visits should be accepted since homeless clients may experience unanticipated changes in their schedules while seeking housing and employment. As crises arise, less frequent, but longer visits may be more successful than many short visits.

Begin at the Beginning   The health care issues of the homeless are multiple and complex. Start with a health issue the client identifies and perceives as less threatening. This may not be the most important need, but it is the client's way of connecting with the provider. Respond to it and move with the client toward more serious issues.

Establish Trust and Respect   Many clients have had unpleasant experiences with the health care system. They look for evidence of the provider's interest, sincerity, and commitment and a relationship that is respectful and trustworthy. They need reassurance that their care will be individualized and focused on what they identify as their needs, even if those needs do not correspond with those assessed by the health care provider. Deliver care to people "where they are" emotionally, physically, and culturally.

Acknowledge Your Client's Culture The cultural norms of the client may not be consistent with the provider's norms. The nurse's expectation of mainstream achievements may be inappropriate for the homeless client. Ask the client about cultural practices. Be sensitive to the client's cultural background and uniqueness and design the intervention around this.

Recognize Obstacles Obstacles may be inherent in the client's lifestyle and it is important to recognize them and work within that context. Issues of safety, shelter, food and economics consume client energy and may place health at a low priority. Low self-esteem or problems perceived by the client as more urgent may result in missed appointments or lack of follow through. Nonjudgmental follow-up strengthens trust and reinforces the nurse's concern for the client. The obstacles to care will become evident and may require a revised plan for intervention.

Identify Learning Styles Many people who are homeless have not been successful in traditional educational settings. Learning how to stay healthy will depend on a presentation based on practical, achievable, behaviors. The provider will need to be persistent and creative to discover educational styles and materials that the client will find relevant and useful.

Provide Social Support Social isolation is common among the homeless. Clients may "somatisize" to fill their need for social interaction. Having someone available to "just listen" often reduces the client's need to make the encounter "problem-focused." Ultimately, this may decrease the isolation and alienation that homeless people describe and improve the success of the health intervention.

Search for Cues Behavior is a method of communication. Recognize and respond appropriately to the nonverbal cues the client is presenting and adjust interventions accordingly.

Advocate!   People who are homeless do not have a collective voice. They generally do not make up a "constituency" in the eyes of their community. Most community members just want the problem of homelessness to be solved. Nurses and other providers of service to the homeless need to assume advocacy roles until the homeless can be empowered as self-advocates.

Collaborate!   Some homeless people avoid involvement with community agencies. Others, particularly children and families, may be working with several service providers. With the client's agreement, discussion with other involved professionals may reveal information that will be of assistance in developing a health promotion plan. Health provider colleagues can support each other in the development of interventions for unfamiliar populations. This support helps to decrease frustration.

Thoughtful consideration must be given to adapting health promotion activities to the circumstances of clients' homelessness. Health professionals should explore living situations with their clients and develop effective plans for nontraditional circumstances. The client's input is essential.

SUMMARY

Nurses may consider it difficult to have an impact on the lifestyle of the homeless. To foster success, nurses must explore their own attitudes toward homelessness, the clients' access to care, methods of adapting care to the life circumstances of individual clients, and the most effective methods of collaborating with other agencies and professionals. Implementation with families and individuals who are homeless will increase the effectiveness of the interactions and make *health promotion*, rather than acute care intervention, a reasonable alternative. Regardless of setting, these suggested strategies for working with homeless clients will benefit nurses and the recipients of their care.

REFERENCES

Berne, A., Dato, C., Mason, D., & Rafferty, M. (1990). A nursing model for addressing the health needs of homeless families. *IMAGE: Journal of Nursing Scholarship*, 22(1), 8–13.

Blau, J. (1992). *The visible poor: Homelessness in the United States.* New York: Oxford University Press.

Elias, C., & Inui, T. (1993). When a house is not a home: Exploring the meaning of shelter among chronically homeless older men. *The Gerontologist, 33*(3), 396–402.

Francis, M. (1992). Eight homeless mothers' tales. *IMAGE: Journal of Nursing Scholarship, 24*(2), 111–114.

Hodnicki, D. (1990). Homelessness: Health care implications. *Journal of Community Health Nursing, 7*(2), 59–67.

McKinney Homeless Assistance Act. (1990). Budget of the United States of America.

United States Department of Health and Human Services. (1992). *Outcasts on Main Street. Report of the Federal Task Force on Homelessness and Severe Mental Illness.* (ADM 92-1904). Washington, DC: Interagency Council on the Homeless.

Ursatine, R., Gelberg, L., Smith, M., & Lesser, J. (1994). Health care for the homeless: A family medicine perspective. *American Family Physician, 49*(1), 139–146.

21

Psychiatric/Mental Health Clinical Experiences in the Community

Challenging Assumptions about the Mentally Ill

Susan Stocker

As nurse educators, one of the most important things we can do to help our students develop critical thinking skills is to challenge their assumptions. A day treatment center for persons who are chronically mentally ill is one of the best places to challenge assumptions about psychiatric clients. The facility we use as a clinical site is a local ambulatory treatment center that offers diagnostic, therapeutic, and rehabilitative services 6 hours per day, 5 days a week. The purpose of this facility is to rehabilitate clients who are chronically mentally ill and to prevent decompensation and the necessity for psychiatric hospitalizations. The clients range in age from 20 to 70 and the most common diagnosis is schizophrenia.

THE CLINICAL EXPERIENCE

The nursing students spend six 3-hour clinical days at the facility. Although they interact with all the clients, the students are assigned a specific client for the duration of their experience. It has been interesting to watch the clients grow as a result of their interactions with the students. One particular client is a favorite of the students. He is a bright young man who grew up in a home where he was abused by his father. When we first started going to the agency, he was assigned to a student. He was always cordial, but when the student mentioned his history of abuse, he would always say, "Let's talk about that next week." Over time, however, he has become more comfortable talking about his childhood experiences. Last fall when another client began to express painful feelings about a personal experience with abuse, this young man was able to provide significant support and guidance to the troubled person. The students spoke afterward about how much the first client had grown, which I believe was in part the result of his experiences with the students. This is an excellent example of two important lessons the students learn from this clinical: the connection between a history of child abuse and the youthful onset of many mental disorders.

The morning is structured to provide at least one group session. A popular one for both students and clients is a support group that is led by staff. Clients sit in a large circle and invite their nursing student to sit beside them. During the support group, there is an informal sharing of issues and concerns. Students are surprised at the clients' knowledge of current events, such as political issues and are impressed with the amount of support offered between clients. Unlike other facilities, where students have been excluded from groups, here they are welcome to participate and support the clients. Although the students have not led this group, they learn about understanding group dynamics and are able to critique the leader's group skills during clinical conference.

OPPORTUNITIES FOR STUDENT LEARNING

Medication Management

Because the facility is staffed by social workers, the clients are responsible for their own medication administration. Clients keep their medications in pill keepers at the facility. The students are surprised at how well informed the clients are about their medications and frequently admit that the clients know more about the medications than they do. Filling the pill keepers gives the students an excellent opportunity to learn about the medications while engaging in a dialogue between themselves and the clients in regard to dosages, side effects, and compliance issues. Because the students are with the clients over several weeks, they become quite skilled in assessing changes in behavior. They can sense when a client may not be taking a medication as prescribed.

Client Teaching

The students come to see each client as more than just someone with a mental illness. Since many of the clients also have physical illnesses, such as diabetes or a seizure disorder, students are able to understand the effects of mental illness on the physical health of the client. Opportunities abound for client teaching in regard to nutrition, exercise, and general health topics.

Planning Group Activities

While the students are at the facility, they are required to lead one activity; this has been a very positive experience. This setting has provided a safe atmosphere for the students to practice the group facilitator role. Faculty provide support and guidance in planning the activity, but the students are responsible for carrying it out with minimal assistance from faculty or staff. Most students plan some type of art or craft activity. At Halloween, clients enjoy painting faces on pumpkins, and at Christmas students help clients make ornaments to decorate the agency tree. One student brought a video camera to the facility and encouraged clients to tell something positive about each other. The session was filmed so that the clients could watch and enjoy the videotape. Other students have led dance or exercise activities. The students have found that the clients often share more openly when they are engaged in an activity, and during this time students are able to make important observations. They assess hand tremors due to medications and escalation of anxiety when clients become frustrated with completion of an activity. They are able to observe how a person approaches activities and how to manage clients who are hallucinating or are severely depressed. The students frequently remark that their participation in activities with the clients is the only time during their hectic week that they are able to exercise or enjoy a relaxing activity themselves. In contrast to the psychiatric clinical horror stories I hear from many seasoned nurses, students frequently remark, "I wish I enjoyed my med-surg clinical as much as this!"

OUTCOMES OF THE EXPERIENCE

Interdisciplinary Focus

Since the agency is staffed by social workers, students are unable to interact with a professional nurse. To compensate, we spend considerable time discussing the potential role of a nurse in this setting. Students are able to differentiate between social work and nursing and are introduced to case management and interdisciplinary services. Students chart on the client's progress notes, and the staff has been impressed with the level of assessment and documentation skills of the nursing students.

Adjacent to the agency there is an office with a registered nurse and a psychiatrist where students have accompanied clients to receive scheduled injections. The nurse has invited students to a group for clients who take Clozaril and she is also available for consultation. After seeing the positive impact of the nurse, students are adamant that the treatment center should also employ a nurse. I encourage them to articulate the benefits of nurses versus other health care providers and to become comfortable "selling themselves" to employers.

Challenging Assumptions

During the clinical experience, students are able to join the clients in activities outside the clinical agency. Everyone enjoys going to the local shopping mall. Students remark how task oriented the clients are and how knowledgeable they are about the stores that offer the best prices and sales. They frequently admit that most of the clients are quicker than they are at determining prices and computing change. Students have noticed how the clients look after and take care of each other. While the feedback about this experience has been overwhelmingly positive, one student came to me at the conclusion of one of our trips to the mall to say that she was nervous about being seen by her acquaintances accompanying a client who is mentally ill. This was a potent reminder that students have assumptions about mental illness and about chronic disabilities that need to be challenged in a supportive environment with peers and faculty.

Students also accompany clients on day trips near Lake Erie. During one outing, I noticed that students were eating very little of the picnic lunch or were taking servings only from dishes their classmates had brought. When questioned, the students expressed concern about the hygienic practices of the clients. Again, students had made assumptions about the mentally ill and were encouraged to challenge those beliefs as the basis for planning sensitive, personalized nursing care.

Over the past few years, the Student Nurses Association has chosen to adopt the entire agency at Christmastime. On a clinical day, the clients decorate ornaments cut out of construction paper and on the opposite side of the ornament, they list items they would like to receive as Christmas gifts. Their humble requests for socks, gloves, and toiletries deeply touch the students who are so aware of our materialistic society. The ornaments are taken to the campus so that all nursing students have the opportunity to select one and purchase a gift for the client. The agency hosts Christmas dinner, which for many of the clients is the only Christmas celebration they will have. Students attend this dinner and are often moved to tears when they see how appreciative the clients are for the gifts. This holiday event has become a tradition that instills good feelings and fond memories of the clinical experience and helps to dispel negative assumptions about the mentally ill.

EVALUATION OF THE EXPERIENCE

This experience is quite different from traditional psychiatric clinical rotations and has consistently been evaluated as valuable and enjoyable. Because the learning experiences in this setting are so unlike those in a traditional setting, faculty must often help students make connections between clinical activities and classroom theory. The students not only learn about psychiatric illness, but also develop many of the skills that are essential in today's rapidly changing health care system: teaching, communicating with individuals and groups, critical thinking, interdisciplinary practice, and caring. Perhaps most importantly, however, students begin to challenge some of their assumptions about the mentally ill and about the reality of living with a chronic illness. Because the students are able to interact with clients in their own personal living environment, not in an institution, the students learn how clients cope on a daily basis. They begin to understand the lived experience of mental illness.

22

A Health Fair for Older Adults

A Community-Based Critical Thinking Activity

Barbara Mc Laughlin
Elaine Bower

The Community College of Philadelphia provides student nurses with a variety of clinical experiences throughout their two-year learning program. In preparing students for the expanding role of the associate degree nurse outside the acute care setting, it is imperative to develop learning opportunities that assist the students to become community focused and appreciate the special health care needs encountered by individuals and families in their homes. The faculty hoped to generate an experience that would enable the students to further develop their critical thinking skills while enhancing their knowledge of the special needs of older adults. A residential continuing care facility for older adults provided an excellent opportunity for associate degree student nurses to enhance their critical thinking skills while exploring and learning about an age-specific population. We were fortunate to have a facility that provided us with access to older adults in all levels of care, independent and assisted living as well as health care. Previously, the primary focus had been with the residents in the health care unit. It became apparent that we were missing learning opportunities in the other areas of the facility.

PLANNING THE HEALTH FAIR

The students, faculty, and residential home health nurses brainstormed about offering a health fair to the residents of the independent and assisted living communities at the facility. With administrative approval, the students used a community-based assessment tool to learn more about resources that were available to all the residents. At the same time, they conducted an assessment to determine specific health care concerns of the residents. They spoke primarily with residents from the independent living community who agreed to be interviewed. Assessment and health education were the primary concerns for the majority of the residents even though many of them believed that they were very healthy in spite of their numerous chronic problems such as diabetes, hypertension, arthritis, and cancers.

The first health fair involved only fourth-semester students. When planning the second health fair, we decided to expand the activity to more than one level of students. Second-semester students were able to assist in the assessment of the population and also in the fair itself. The two levels of students, working together, provided opportunities to enhance leadership and role-modeling skills for both groups. In addition to the benefits for the residents, the students thoroughly enjoyed working together on a project and seeing the successful end results. They were the envy of the Community College of Philadelphia Nursing program. Up until this time, second-semester students had spent much of their time with ill older adults in acute care settings. This health fair allowed them to work with older adults in their home/community setting. In planning and executing the health fair, both students and the faculty experienced discovery learning and focused inquiry.

The development of the students' collaborative skills was enhanced through interaction with key people within the facility. It was necessary for the students to meet with these key people to work out the nitty-gritty details of the health fair. Preliminary interaction between the faculty and the key individuals set the groundwork for the students. Students were to learn the role that each person or department would play in organizing and presenting the health fair. Although the nursing faculty was readily available for support and problem-solving, it was the students' responsibility to make appointments with the appropriate person. This was an excellent opportunity as it involved interactions with people in the everyday workings of the facility. Some of these key people included the administrator, director of nursing, social service, public relations, maintenance, food services, activities personnel, nurses in the medical offices and representatives to the resident council. All of them were very receptive to students' requests for information. Knowing which key person to call was especially helpful when problems arose on the day of the event. As a result of this ongoing collaboration, the health fair was received with great enthusiasm, and the students recognized that identifying and involving key people was a significant factor in the successful completion of their project. We found that encouraging this interaction from the beginning of the project enhanced the quality of the entire clinical experience.

Planning and carrying out a health fair is a creative process that involves much more than nursing knowledge. Both students and faculty learned that there were many aspects to making the event a success besides a working knowledge of every antihypertensive known to the medical profession. As a result of our first health fair we learned that food and flexibility were elements that could not be ignored. These two factors became cornerstones in the implementation of the health fair.

OFFERINGS AT THE HEALTH FAIR

After completing the community assessment, all of the students met together to decide the offerings for the health fair and to divide up the tasks. Each work group involved both levels of students and faculty. In addition to blood pressure and weight screening, the students decided to provide medication reviews and information on nutrition and safety.

All these activities provided the students with ample opportunity to build on their teaching skills since they needed to look at the special needs of the older adults and plan their presentations accordingly. Hearing and vision deficits provided special challenges, from designing posters and handouts to actually communicating effectively with the residents.

Screenings

From our first health fair we realized that residents frequently requested blood pressure measurements and weights. These skills are easy to perform and both levels of students could be involved. The resident was then given a record of the blood pressure and weight for future comparison. Residents with abnormal blood pressure readings were referred to the in-house wellness nurse for follow-up.

Many residents requested blood sugar and cholesterol screening. Even though students are prepared to perform the necessary finger sticks and the tests for blood sugar and cholesterol screening, legal ramifications must be addressed prior to performing these invasive procedures. Also inaccurate test results, especially for blood sugars, may occur depending on the time the blood sample is collected in relation to meals or snacks ingested. This has the potential for raising unnecessary concern in the mind of the resident.

Medication Review

Critical thinking skills were constantly being strengthened throughout this exercise. Once the tasks were divided, research and content selection required a great deal of thought and consideration. Since the students could not possibly look up every medication, they needed to determine which ones this population used most frequently. Through interviews and assessment, the students developed a list of the most common medications and familiarized themselves with those. They also brought several drug handbooks with them to the fair. The students discovered that many of the older adults who attended our fair were remarkably well informed about their medications but were still eager to learn anything new that the students might be able to tell them.

In conjunction with the medication assessment, the students helped the resident update the emergency medical information card that each resident is asked to place on the inside of his or her apartment door. Many of these cards had not been updated in some time. This required the students to ask focused questions and to interpret and record the responses accurately.

Safety Education

Older adults tend to have a greater number of injuries than the general population as a result of accidents in the home. Therefore, during our first health fair, we decided to perform a home safety assessment for the residents at the long-term care facility. Two students researched a number of available tools and then developed one of their own that would provide a basis for teaching the residents how to avoid injuries in their apartments (Figure 22–1). The original plan was for the student to actually walk through the apartment with the resident and together, do the assessment. Because of hesitancy on the part of the residents, we handed out the assessments and spoke with each resident who took one. In review, we realized that privacy and creative home adaptations were

Figure 22–1
Home Safety Checklist

	Yes	No
All Areas—Check Cords		
Are lamp, extension, and telephone cords placed out of the flow of traffic?	___	___
Are cords out from beneath furniture legs and rugs/carpeting?	___	___
Are cords attached to the walls with nails or staples?	___	___
Are electrical cords in good condition, not frayed or cracked?	___	___
Check all Rugs, Runners, Mats		
Are all small rugs, runners, and mats slip-resistant?	___	___
Telephone Area		
Are emergency numbers posted on or near the telephone?	___	___
Do you have access to a telephone if you fall (accessible if you are unable to stand)?	___	___
Electrical Outlets and Switches		
Are any outlets or switches unusually warm or hot to the touch?	___	___
Do all outlets and switches have cover plates so that no wiring is exposed?	___	___
Check lightbulbs		
Are lightbulbs the appropriate size and type for the lamp or fixture (if unknown—use a maximum of 60 watts)?	___	___
Check Smoke Detectors		
Do you have properly working smoke detectors?	___	___
Kitchen		
Are towels and curtains located away from the range?	___	___
Are extension cords and appliance cords located away from the sink and range areas?	___	___
Hallways		
Are hallways and passageways between rooms well lit?	___	___
Are exits and passageways kept clear?	___	___
Bathrooms		
Are bathtubs and showers equipped with nonskid mats, abrasive, or nonslippery surfaces?	___	___
Do bathtubs and showers have grab bars?	___	___
Medications		
Are all medicines stored in the original containers and clearly marked?	___	___
Bedrooms		
Are lamps or light switches within the reach of the bed?	___	___
Is there a telephone close to the bed?	___	___

Note: Developed by Kenneth O'Brien, SN, CCP, Class of 1995.

carefully guarded by all the residents. During our second health fair, we again used the home safety assessment tool but did not offer to go with the resident to complete the assessment. Instead the students reviewed the plan with the residents and encouraged them to do it on their own. The residents were very receptive to this approach. The student also created posters and handouts with safety tips.

Since much of our population was very mobile and continued to drive and use public transportation, safety was a real issue. In preparation, the students explored and contacted several outside resources that offered safety tips for the elderly. Our local police department offered to present a program on personal safety.

Nutrition

In keeping with our healthy theme, faculty and students explored many sources for recipes that were low fat, low cholesterol, sugar-free, and low sodium. They also had to be tasty and easy to prepare. We learned from our first experience that the foods had to be portable and easy to eat. Students prepared and served samples of these foods. These snacks were placed at various booths throughout the fair to prevent any one area from becoming too congested as residents and staff quickly gravitated to the food. Several students created large posters depicting nutritional information as well as handouts for the residents. This provided an additional opportunity for interaction between students and residents. Copies of these easy-to-prepare recipes were available for the residents and staff to take and try on their own. The facility generously provided a fruit tray as well as coffee and tea. A local bakery donated low-fat pastries and a pretzel bakery donated salt-free soft pretzels. Our college bookstore provided bags for carrying samples and handouts (and perhaps a snack for later); the bags also reminded the residents which school was presenting the fair.

During our first fair, we were able to obtain samples of nutritional liquid supplements. The students were excited about this but the residents seemed less than willing to try the samples or take the coupons and free cans of the supplement. They did however, take the pamphlets on nutrition. This leads us to believe that the residents were afraid others would think they were ill or unable to eat properly if they were seen taking the supplement. There is great concern for preserving one's independence in continuing care communities and the residents take pains to protect themselves.

Resources

In spite of the lack of interest in the nutritional supplements, it is a good idea to contact pharmaceutical companies as well as other suppliers and local merchants for help. They are excellent resources for samples and "giveaways." One student visited a local plant nursery and received a donation of several plants that were used to adorn the various booths and later were awarded as door prizes. These plants were presented to the winners while they were having their lunch in the dining room much to the delight of all those who had attended the health fair.

KEY COMPONENTS OF THE HEALTH FAIR

Flexibility

Our first health fair taught us the necessity of flexibility. Despite careful planning, on the morning of the health fair we had to move to three different locations with two different sets of tables. Much to our advantage, the final location was an ideal setting, just outside the main dining room. Every resident and employee knew where the dining room was located. This area is convenient and accessible to all residents and employees. Attendance was excellent. This validates the importance of location, location, location! Because of this location, employees were also able to bring some residents from the health care units to the fair. This was particularly gratifying since the students spend most of their time with this group of people. In addition, the employees were able to take advantage of the information, screening, and samples at the health fair. This contributed to a continuing cooperative relationship with the staff of the health care unit. We, of course, requested this same location for our second health fair.

Student assignments also required considerable flexibility. While each student prepared to be an expert in a certain area, it was often necessary for a student to assist in another area when it became busy. Second- and fourth-semester students were paired and moved together. It was important for students to be able to take the time to talk with residents and answer their questions completely and in an unhurried manner. Each one needed to be aware of everyone else and move freely from one place to another. This required familiarity with the total situation by all the students involved the day of the fair. The students developed a great deal of confidence from being able to speak intelligently on a variety of subjects. Faculty and fourth-semester students had many opportunities for role-modeling communication and problem-solving skills.

Timing

The timing of the health fair is another important factor and requires some flexibility on the part of both faculty and students as well as the facility. It is important to plan the fair for days when other activities are not occurring at the facility. We were careful to check the posted calendar for bus trips and shopping trips as well as clearing our plans with the activities personnel. Because we were located in a self-contained continuing care community, weather was not a problem. This would, however, be an issue if participants were traveling to a senior center or other location. It may be necessary for the faculty and the facility to select a day well in advance of actual student participation. Some adjustments needed to be made regarding clinical days and times with compromises from both groups of students. Clinical days were changed to permit students to do the community and needs assessment several weeks in advance of the date selected for the health fair. It is also best to check with the facility about the time of day. Because we were offering food samples, we wanted to be sure not to disrupt meals or special dietary plans. The event was scheduled for three hours in the morning so as not to interfere with regularly scheduled afternoon activities.

Public Relations

Public relations, social service, and individuals from the resident council were very helpful in advertising the health fair. Advance notification of the health fair appeared in the in-house monthly newsletter. The students prepared a flyer with all the necessary information. This was then distributed by volunteers to each apartment and room throughout independent and assisted living areas. Posters were placed on the bulletin boards. Announcements were made in chapel and over the in-house television station. "We'll see you at the Health Fair" was frequently heard as students talked with residents.

OUTCOMES OF THE HEALTH FAIR

All the residents thoroughly enjoyed interacting with the students, while the students learned a great deal about them. Approximately 150 students, faculty, residents, and staff participated in the first health fair. By the second year, more than 200 people attended, and the outcomes far exceeded the original expectations. The students became quite comfortable with the residents and the residential setting while learning about the special needs and adaptability of the geriatric population. Additional benefits included the enhancement of the following student skills: organization and planning, assessment and observation, communications and interviewing, teaching, medications, and adaptability. Students participated in this activity with renewed energy and enthusiasm.

Planning and presenting a health fair requires that the faculty look beyond the confines of the acute care setting or the nursing home to identify and provide new and challenging learning experiences. It provides an opportunity for the faculty to observe students interacting in group activities, leadership roles, and decision-making exercises. The health fair is an experience with endless creative possibilities. The faculty and students challenged one another in devising varied learning situations. Everyone had the chance to learn, often by trial and error. Constructive criticism and "let's try it and see" approaches were key survival techniques for both faculty and students.

The faculty and students met immediately after the event to critique the activity. Each person was asked to make a suggestion about his or her area for future events. We discussed both positive and negative factors as well as things to keep and things to change. This was a semistructured conference that ended our day on a high note. Ideally, we hope that our second-semester participants will be able to serve as leaders for future health fairs at this facility, thereby providing continuity.

We would be remiss if we led anyone to believe that everything went like clockwork in the planning and implementation of these health fairs. However, it is from our mistakes that we learn the most. For example, we advertised the medication assessment the first year as "brown bag" medication review. The students and faculty knew what this meant, but the residents thought that we were inviting them to talk with us about their medications over a lunch provided by us! None of them brought their medications with them.

Figure 22-2
Top Ten Tips to Remember When Planning a Health Fair in a Community-Based Setting with an Older Adult Population

1. Location, Location, Location! Try to situate the health fair on the route to or from some essential activity (e.g., the dining room).
2. Have plenty of mobile help—people who are available to listen uninterrupted to the older adult.
3. Food is always a major draw. It should be easy to eat and also portable. They love to pack it away for later. Coffee is a must!
4. Plan well in advance—pick a day when there are no bus trips or shopping excursions.
5. Be flexible with your setup. Regulations sometimes dictate which chairs, tables, rooms, and other equipment you can use.
6. Include the staff. Be sure to make them feel welcome. Offer to take blood pressures.
7. Communicate fully and frequently with appropriate key people (administrators, public relations, resident representatives, etc.).
8. Publicize early and in a variety of ways.
9. Tap outside resources—local merchants, pharmaceutical representatives.
10. Have a good sense of humor. Keep Murphy's Law in mind—Whatever can go wrong, will go wrong.

FUTURE PLANS

We plan to continue this health fair on an annual basis at this facility, building on what we learn each year. We also hope to involve students in health fairs at a variety of other locations throughout the community and with other age groups. Each time we participate in planning and presenting one of these events, we expand our knowledge of available resources as well as promote the health and safety of the target populations.

Off the record, if you are a faculty member and planning a health fair (see Figure 22-2), remember to keep your sense of humor and be flexible.

23

Pediatric Health Fairs in Elementary Schools and Community Settings

Ann Marie LaMarca Major
Barbara B. Marckx
Michelle Codner

With the implementation of managed care, the philosophy of health care delivery has dramatically shifted from an acute care climate where interventions were focused on secondary and tertiary levels of prevention to a community environment where the emphasis is on primary prevention. On a national level, in the Pew Commission report, nursing programs have been called on to carefully assess the competencies of their graduates and to apply these assessments to redefine the core of their curricula (Shugars, O'Neil, & Bader, 1991). On a professional level, nursing education programs need to ensure that all nurses are prepared to function in a community-focused health care system (National League for Nursing, 1993).

This evolution in health care challenges nursing education programs to develop alternative educational strategies. With the movement of the client population into the community, hospital clinical experiences for students, especially in the area of pediatrics, are insufficient and are at an acuity level well beyond the scope of the student. Driven by these trends, a community-focused pediatric clinical nursing project was developed. The pediatric health fair project is consistent with the educational objectives set forth by both the Pew Commission and the National League for Nursing. The project addresses community health needs and develops critical thinking skills through a learning strategy based on the concept of primary prevention for the pediatric population. Table 23–1 shows the outline followed to implement this project.

Table 23–1
Outline for Implementation of Pediatric Health Fair

I. Planning
  A. Assessment of community organizations involved in the care/education of children to determine:
    1. Health promotion programs available.
    2. Additional needs for health promotion education.
    3. Community organizations' interest in participation.
  B. Collaborative planning between college and organization:
    1. Meeting to clarify project parameters—
      a. Date and time of event.
      b. Physical environment for the fair.
      c. Children's schedule.
      d. Nursing students' responsibilities.
    2. Develop letter of agreement.
  C. Preparation of Nursing Students:
    1. Development of student guidelines.
    2. Guidance related to learning materials/equipment.
II. Implementation
  A. Setup of materials and equipment at fair site.
  B. Supervision of health fair activities.
III. Evaluation
  A. Postconference discussion and evaluation.
  B. Written evaluation by students and organization.
  C. Revision of project based on evaluation data.

CURRICULUM

The curricular focus of the pediatric health fair project was on the creation of a student clinical experience that matched changing trends in health care delivery to the needs of the pediatric population in the community. Key concepts integrated into this experience included fundamentals of growth and development, primary prevention in the pediatric population, and principles of teaching/learning theory.

    The pediatric health fair pilot project was integrated into the clinical curriculum for Broome Community College's nursing students during the third or fourth semester of the program. In cooperation with community agencies, the students were given an assignment to create and implement a health fair for children. This pediatric community experience comprised one clinical day.

COMMUNITY ASSESSMENT

The community assessment phase of the project was conducted by the pediatric nursing faculty. Organizations that offered programs for children including the YMCA, Head Start, the Urban League, and local school districts were assessed to determine their interest in a collaborative health promotion project with the Broome Community College (BCC) nursing program. Once interest in the project was determined, nursing faculty met with community organization administrators to review the health promotion programs that were in place and determine how to incorporate the health fair format into these programs. A contract, in the form of a letter, clarified the roles of the parties involved. Additional meetings were held to work out the fine points of the project such as date and time, environmental needs (tables, electrical outlets, wall space, etc.), and schedules for movement of the children through the health fair.

PROJECT IMPLEMENTATION

The first community site chosen for BCC nursing students to implement the pediatric health fair project was a local elementary school with a population of 350 children ranging in age from 5 through 11 years. Nursing faculty met with the principal of the school to develop a handout for teachers that explained the project and a schedule for circulating the children through the health fair. The role of the teachers was to remain with their classes and to help maintain order during the health fair. Resources recommended to the teachers to help prepare the children for the health fair included books, such as *The Magic School Bus: Inside the Human Body*, and the film *The Incredible Journey*.

Nursing faculty designed guidelines for the clinical experience that required the students to use critical thinking skills to develop learning stations for the children. The concepts of growth and developmental theory, primary prevention for the pediatric client, and teaching/learning theory were to be integrated into each learning situation. Creativity was encouraged with recommendations for the development of learning materials (coloring pages, word puzzles), skits, and audiovisual presentations that would enhance the learning process.

Eighteen nursing students participated in the health fair pilot project. They were divided into four groups with each group required to develop a learning station to present to the children. Nursing instructors were available for consultation and guidance, but students were responsible for their own lesson plans and materials. The students were encouraged to network with local chapters of the American Heart Association and the American Cancer Society for assistance with audiovisual aids and learning tools. The college copy center was available to students, as needed, as was a budget of one hundred dollars for the purchase of paper, supplies, and decorations.

The elementary school made the gymnasium and cafeteria available for the morning sessions of the health fair. The cafeteria was set up with learning stations for the children in kindergarten through second grade. Learning stations for third through fifth graders were set up in the gymnasium. While the topics for the stations were the same for kindergarten through fifth-grade students, it was important to use different environments because teaching methods were tailored to meet the different developmental levels.

The nursing students chose the following topics for the learning stations: "How We Stay Well," "First Aid for Bleeding and Bones," "How Our Lungs Work," and "A Visit to the Hospital." Stations, colorfully decorated with balloons and posters, provided hands-on experiences to gain the interest of the children. The nursing students incorporated teaching strategies based on the psychological and developmental concepts of Erikson and Piaget. For children in the 5- to 7-year age group, dolls and stuffed animals served as "patients" at the "Visit to the Hospital" learning station. Children could handle stethoscopes, gloves, and masks. Blood pressures were taken and ear thermometers were demonstrated by a nursing student wearing a clown costume. A student dressed as Minnie Mouse measured weight and stature.

For children 8 to 11 years in age, skeletons were on display for identifying the bones of the body and illustrating how injury occurs. Students demonstrated the use of splints and elastic bandages with child volunteers. Bacteria grown on agar plates reinforced the concept of germs and led into the topic of proper hand washing for control of such germs.

Children learned how their lungs work and about the dangers of smoking. Each learning station provided a creative, developmentally appropriate opportunity to learn about primary prevention.

OUTCOMES

Nursing faculty evaluated each learning station and student presentation. The responses of children to the learning activities made it evident to faculty that the nursing students had used critical thinking skills in the preparation and implementation of their projects. Faculty noted that many of the students who had been insecure in the acute care clinical area were effective teachers of children in the community setting.

In addition, faculty used a postconference format to discuss and evaluate the clinical experience. This conference gave the nursing students a forum to analyze the effectiveness of their presentations and to revise their teaching plans. Overall, students reported that the experience was valuable and enhanced their understanding of growth and developmental theory, pediatric primary prevention, and teaching/learning theory.

Written evaluation of the project was done with a questionnaire distributed to nursing students, teachers, and school administrators. Response was enthusiastic and included suggestions for future health fairs. Recommendations noted the need to control for noise. The choice of gymnasium for a presentation environment was less than optimal because of acoustic problems with a large number of children in one room. Use of individual classrooms for learning stations could eliminate this problem.

The elementary school teachers were a valuable asset in helping to move the children through each learning station and in keeping the environment well controlled for effective learning. One group of teachers suggested that the children be encouraged to make posters about health to be used as decorations at the health fair.

EXPANSION OF THE PROJECT

Following the initial project, the Department of Nursing received inquiries from four other elementary schools interested in collaborating with BCC. Based on the overall success of the pilot project, BCC has integrated the pediatric health fair project into its community-focused curriculum (see Chapter 11, Marckx & Denman). In addition to fairs at elementary schools during the school hours, the Department of Nursing has collaborated with community organizations to offer pediatric health fairs during Parents' Night school programs, YMCA "Healthy Kids' Day," and various day-care programs throughout the community.

The campus community as a whole has become energized and taken an active interest in the project. BCC's Campus Day Care Center sponsored a pediatric health fair in which the children, ranging in age from 2 to 4 years, and their preschool teachers were guests at the nursing learning laboratory. A pediatric health fair component was even incorporated into the 50th-anniversary celebration of the college.

SUMMARY

The pediatric health fair project is an innovative learning strategy that has challenged nursing students' critical thinking abilities. By designing and implementing creative activities for children, the students have learned to synthesize and apply concepts of growth and developmental theory, pediatric primary prevention, and the teaching/learning process. The pediatric health fair project has been effective in building strong relationships with community organizations and has enhanced community-focused nursing care.

REFERENCES

National League for Nursing. (1993). *A vision for nursing education.* National League for Nursing Position Paper. New York: Author.

Shugars, D. A., O'Neil, E. H., & Bader, J. D. (1991). *Healthy America: Practitioners for 2005, an agenda for action for U.S. health professional schools.* Durham, NC: Pew Health Professions Commission.

24

Family-Centered Community Care in a Rural Setting

Sue A. Wise
Jacqueline Watercutter

Edison Community College is located in rural, southwestern Ohio. The associate degree nursing program has a long history of following clients as they move from hospital to community settings and preparing nurses to care for them. The nursing faculty introduce community concepts and experiences throughout the program with increasing depth of involvement. Students spend one-half of their final semester in Family-Centered Community Care (FCCC). FCCC is one-half of the capstone course of the nursing program. The content is Pediatrics, which works well for the community focus. We are able to use the family as client in a variety of integrated settings. FCCC is an autonomous experience for the students, requiring them to negotiate to creatively solve problems and collaborate independently with health care colleagues in the community. Students are responsible for their schedules, within guidelines, and every reasonable effort is made to allow students to identify and fill their own needs as they come to the end of the nursing program.

PROGRAM DEVELOPMENT

Focus Groups

Focus groups of community health care professionals have helped immeasurably to build FCCC. Focus group data identified needs in our community that could be satisfied by our students while meeting program

271

outcomes. School nurses explained new mandatory health teaching curriculum requirements. Teachers, it was reported, often do not have time or expertise to prepare the lessons, and school nurses are overwhelmed by mandated screenings and increasing crisis intervention to do this teaching. Assistance is needed at health fairs for children due to increasing cutbacks in area hospital budgets for this type of outreach assistance. Head Start managers reported needing help with nutritional screening and teaching to meet state requirements.

Marketing

We have found that the development and maintenance of relationships with nurse colleagues in the community is vital. Marketing (finding needs and filling them) is the key to our success in identifying and maintaining optimum clinical opportunities for our students in these competitive times. We asked these questions: "Where are the children with needs?" "How can we meet those needs while meeting student learning needs?" We applied basic marketing principles in developing relationships with community preceptors. Frequent meetings, lunches, and ongoing dialogue on a year-round basis have resulted in strong, committed relationships, positive student experiences, and employment of graduates. One example is our county hospice unit, which has hired two new graduates in a newly developed internship program. Both nurses are now functioning as full-time staff members. A local family practice asked for applications from graduates who had spent FCCC clinical time in their office and hired a new graduate.

Administrative Support

Administrative support cannot be overestimated in the development of FCCC. An administrator with a prudent, risk-taking perspective, who visualizes the future of health care delivery, is the foundation from which FCCC grew. Financial as well as moral support fostered the ongoing development of this undertaking.

PROJECT IMPLEMENTATION

Projects have and are being developed by students and faculty to meet these needs in cooperation with our community colleagues. Resulting assignments allow students to assess, compare, and interact with children of various ages and developmental stages. Preparation of age-appropriate teaching materials and collaboration with children, families, and community colleagues in holistic ways are highlights of FCCC. The interactive class assignments allow students to develop autonomy and creatively meet program outcomes. The vision of the community college as a community resource is enhanced by the relationships developed by the nursing faculty and students with FCCC.

Students are valuable resources for families in the community. As students develop a family-community perspective along with increasing autonomy, they are encouraged to plan clinical experiences that meet their individual interests and career goals within the structure of the course. To meet program outcomes, students explore areas of particular interest to them. Examples include health teaching in a battered women's shelter, interacting with a children's services caseworker to identify creative ways for nurses to help families in crisis, and spending a day in a burn unit.

Sites and Schedules

Individual schedules are provided to students several weeks before the 8-week FCCC rotation. Flexibility is required of students, although an effort is made to give advance notice to students for child care and work arrangements.

There are now 20 clinical sites. Student clinical experiences are not identified and are not observational. Individual schedules provide each student with a variety of clinical experiences, such as screening and educational settings for mentally retarded children, clinics, family practices, pediatrician offices, schools, Head Start, urgent care, nurse phone referral, and community teaching projects.

The first 10 clinical hours are spent on campus with growth and development and community concepts. Sequential experiences in a clinical site are provided where appropriate.

Evaluation

Instructors are available by beeper to students and preceptors. Site visits are made by instructors periodically for student evaluation and interaction with preceptors. Students are given clinical evaluation forms weekly on which they are asked to evaluate each clinical experience, list skills practiced at each site and give suggestions for improvement. Based on evaluations, clinical experiences are expanded or discontinued.

Preceptors

Clinical preceptors give feedback to students and instructors on student performance as well as ongoing suggestions for improvement of FCCC. Faculty meet with preceptors again at the end of the semester for discussion regarding changes or improvements that can be made for the following year. We have been continually heartened by the acceptance and assistance of our nurse colleagues in the community. Their comments have been consistent with ours in the process of student performance. Development of schedules that allow students to plan clinical times with the same nurse rather than with a clinical site has resulted in increased opportunities to practice skills. The student develops rapport with the preceptor and can demonstrate competence over several days, resulting in increased practice of hands-on nursing skills. Clinical preceptors receive personal thank-you letters from the faculty at the end of each semester.

Student Care Conferences

FCCC culminates with a Student Care Conference during the final clinical week. The care conference is an all-inclusive postconference designed to allow all students to benefit from the clinical experience of each student. Brochures are printed, and preceptors as well as interested college and community people are invited to attend. The Care Conference begins with a carefully chosen speaker, who has community and family expertise. A panel of recent graduate nurses who work in nontraditional settings follows the speaker. They describe their work settings and answer questions from students. Pairs of students are responsible for 40-minute presentations describing a pertinent research-based topic applied to a selected clinical experience. Peer evaluation is conducted by the students.

PILOT PROJECT

A pilot program was implemented during the summer of 1996. Camp Courageous is a hospice-run camp for children aged 5 to 18 who have suffered the loss of a significant other. The county hospice nurses and social workers were enthusiastic about implementing a pilot program with Edison Community College using nursing students in their final semester. The day camp was one week in length. The pilot program was designed to allow students to work with children with needs in community settings and bank clinical time before the FCCC rotation. Students applied for the pilot program in large numbers. Ten students were randomly selected. The students sent an application to Camp Courageous personnel, were interviewed and took part in a hospice training session. Students further prepared by reviewing growth, development, and bereavement materials selected by faculty from the syllabus used for the FCCC course.

Students attended the full week of day camp. Hospice nurses, social workers, and chaplains were present at the camp. Journals were kept regarding time spent, daily activities, interactions with children, developmental stage, grief process, and suggestions for improving the experience. Students took part in an oral discussion with faculty after returning to campus for fall semester. Students spent approximately 40 to 45 clock hours with Camp Courageous. A postcamp staff meeting was included in the time as well as a camp reunion in September 1996.

Students are credited for clinical time based on FCCC course outcomes met by the Camp Courageous experience. Students must attend a campus lab on growth and development and community concepts to begin the FCCC course. They must spend two full clinical days in one additional clinical site. These experiences allow students to prepare for and take part in the Student Care Conference, which is the culmination of FCCC.

To allow for in-depth interactions, students were assigned as personal companions for one to three children. In addition, students were assigned to a group of children of the same age range for group activities. Activities were structured to begin and end with play alternating with periods of bereavement work. A memory book was completed by each child. Arts, crafts, nature walks, music, and swimming were included in the schedule. Children wrote poetry and drew family portraits. Questions were presented to nurses at group discussions (e.g., "What if the ambulance came sooner?", "How does cancer work?"). Camp Courageous closed with a memorial service. Children made ornaments that were hung on a tree. Songs and poetry were presented by the children, and family members attended the event.

The oral discussion with student participants has led us to redesign our Camp Courageous preparation materials. We will include a review of therapeutic communication techniques and an expectation of deeper study of growth and development concepts pertinent to specific age groups assigned to each student. Hospice training for students focuses on bereavement so we are eliminating that piece from our preparation.

Further changes may be made for next year pending review of student journals and a discussion with hospice personnel. Students unanimously reported the Camp Courageous pilot was a valuable clinical experience. A few students thought the camp should be mandatory for all students. A meeting will take place between faculty and hospice staff to further allow us to evaluate the Camp Courageous experience. A letter received from hospice personnel expressed a very positive reaction to the program and a desire to repeat it. Specific objectives for the experience are being developed based on final evaluation of the pilot.

Based on the final evaluation of Camp Courageous as a clinical experience for FCCC, we will explore other similar summer camps for children with needs (camps would include children with diabetes, developmental delays, cancer, and neuromuscular diseases). We are excited by opportunities that provide experience with children and allow us to meet needs in our role as a community college.

FUTURE PLANS

Future plans include a nutrition screening project for Head Start to begin in spring 1997. This project will target children within a Head Start program (infancy to school age). The nursing students will utilize a comprehensive tool that evaluates various elements with regard to child development and nutrition. Critical thinking skills will be utilized as the student takes the data and collaborates with the nutritionist, social worker, on-site RN, and faculty for a referral or ongoing plan of care. This pilot project was developed based on feedback received from data collected in the focus groups held in the spring 1996. This project is planned for implementation for spring 1997. Future focus groups will be held with graduates from our program to further refine FCCC. In addition, we are considering provision of continuing education credit for the Student Care Conference. We plan to develop product offerings to meet needs identified in focus groups. The products would consist of research-based, consistently implemented programs such as bicycle safety, first aid leveled for various ages, and basic hygiene for caregivers of Head Start children. These workshops will address community needs as well as meet FCCC program outcomes.

Based on the support we have received from our administration and the positive evaluative data we have gathered, we look forward to growing our Family-Centered Community Care course to further benefit our students, our college, and our community.

25

A Collaborative Project to Provide Primary Health Care in Schools

Ruth A. DePalma

BACKGROUND INFORMATION

The Educational Alliance of Pueblo, Colorado, a partnership between Pueblo School District No. 60 and the University of Southern Colorado, aspires to strengthen the quality of education from elementary through higher education (Grades K-16). This is accomplished through the combining of resources, so financial savings can be channeled into classroom improvements and partnerships to achieve academic needs at both institutions.

Administrators, faculty, and staff in School District No. 60 and the University of Southern Colorado Department of Nursing were concerned about the health of all individuals, especially those who do not have and/or have difficulty accessing or receiving health care services. Both organizations were also concerned about the knowledge and understanding of health issues within the community and among all levels of students, especially since the school district was without nursing services. Educators and parents were aware of the relationships between a healthy child and literacy, literacy and a future, the future of individuals and the hope of a community.

Information from the Colorado Department of Health and Pueblo School District No. 60 indicated that some of its schoolchildren might be experiencing attendance and learning difficulties due to health-related needs. Community interest and support for improving the health care of children were evident, but activities initiated by various community groups resulted in fragmentation, duplication, or gaps in essential health services.

With the nationwide shift in health care from acute settings to the community, it is predicted the demand for nurses in the community will continue to rise. Nursing programs are going through curriculum revision to focus on community-based care. Schools are ideal settings for community-focused care. It was determined that students enrolled in the Nursing Program at the University of Southern Colorado would benefit from learning experiences with well children and community-based efforts in the schools. They needed opportunities to participate in health assessments, health promotion and teaching, and primary health care of children and families. Faculty would also benefit from the Alliance through opportunities for research studies and clinical practice. The district's need for nursing services and the University of Southern Colorado's need for community health and pediatric nursing experiences were the impetus for the Education Alliance of Pueblo Nursing Partnership.

ESTABLISHING A PARTNERSHIP

After much negotiation between the College Dean, University of Southern Colorado administrators, and the chair of the Nursing Program, it was decided to form a partnership for nursing. The coordinator of this program is a master's or PhD prepared registered nurse who teaches half-time at the University of Southern Colorado in the Department of Nursing and serves half-time in School District No. 60 as nursing services coordinator. This nurse is responsible for:

- Strengthening the school health program through collaboration with the Health Education Specialist in Pueblo School District No. 60 to examine, evaluate, advise, promote, and strengthen health services for children in the district.
- Planning and organizing a practicum/clinical arena for University of Southern Colorado nursing students, allowing them to develop a better understanding of the health needs of school-age children and community-based care while practicing nursing related to health education and health promotion.
- Program Evaluation, both formative and summative, to determine the effectiveness of the nursing partnership.

Each partner contributes 50 percent of salary and benefits for this position. The actual contract is a University tenure-track position. In the original proposal, responsibilities specific to Pueblo School District No. 60 and University of Southern Colorado Department of Nursing were specified but unrealistic in scope. Prioritization narrowed down these responsibilities to more realistic expectations. Otherwise, the halves of the partnership could easily have been converted into two full-time loads for the nurse coordinator.

Expected goals and outcomes as a result of the nursing partnership, which were identified and met within the first two years of the project and continue to be expanded, are identified in Table 25–1.

Table 25–1
Project Outcomes

1. Analysis of a Needs Assessment that identified health needs (and geographic pockets of those needs) of children attending Pueblo School District No. 60 schools.
2. Establishment of a comprehensive School Health Education Council that provides guidance and input into school health issues.
3. Coordination of screening activities and improved follow-up of children with vision and hearing deficiencies.
4. Computerization of student health records (vision, hearing, immunizations, medications, and health problems).
5. Establishment of clinical practicums/laboratories for University of Southern Colorado nursing students that provide:
   a. Learning activities for University of Southern Colorado students.
   b. Additional health education/information for District No. 60 students.
   c. Additional health services for children attending District No. 60 schools.
   d. Home visits for children at risk.
   e. Education of teachers and staff related to health problems presented in the classroom.
6. Development of staff wellness programs.
7. Implementation of nursing delegation for medication administration in the schools.
8. Development of a paid pool of senior nursing students for head lice screening and follow-up.
9. Formative and summative evaluation.

STUDENT EXPERIENCES AND NURSE COORDINATOR ACTIVITIES

From involvement with this partnership, the nurse coordinator changed student experiences in the pediatric and community health nursing courses, linking nursing students with school district, students, and staff. Student experiences for which the coordinator provides specific guidelines are listed in Table 25–2. Activities of the nurse coordinator, including school district responsibilities and academic responsibilities are included in Table 25–3.

Health and school district information is readily accessible to the coordinator for follow-up of health concerns or screenings. Because the schools are familiar with the program, the coordinator has rapid access to the schools for planned and unplanned student experiences. If the

Table 25–2
Student Experiences and Objectives

Vision/hearing screening and follow-up.

Scoliosis screening.

Home visits to high-risk families/family assessment.

Immunization record review and follow-up.

Community needs assessment.

Health education and promotion activities.

Staff health fairs and in-services.

Growth and development projects.

Identification of health needs of school-age children.

Head lice identification and follow-up.

Communicable disease follow-up.

Involvement in research projects.

Coordination with community agencies/boards that provide services to the school district.

Teaching basic hygiene skills to children and families.

Evaluating comprehensive health education.

Interaction with special needs children.

Preschool physicals.

Immunization clinics.

Epidemiology.

Table 25–3
Activities of the Nurse-Coordinator

School District Responsibilities

Collaboration with District No. 60 Health Education Specialist on Comprehensive School Health Education and other community related programs.

Coordination of vision and hearing screenings.

Coordination of immunization records.

Computerization of screening and immunization records.

Home visits to high-risk families/collaboration with social services.

Head lice identification follow-up.

Coordination of immunization clinics.

Staff wellness programs/in-services.

Resource for District No. 60 administration and school on issues related to health/ nursing.

Medication delegation classes and consultation.

Needs assessments.

Consultation with the State School Nursing Specialist.

Membership on various advisory/community boards.

Academic Responsibilities

Teaching six credit hours at the university each semester.

Coordination and placement of students in the schools and community settings.

University and Department functions/committees.

Coordination of pediatric and community health courses.

Attendance at committee meetings and conferences related to school nursing.

Presentations concerning the Alliance Nursing Partnership.

Position evaluation.

coordinator of this program were not an official employee of the school district as well as the university, many opportunities for student experiences would not be possible. For example, when one of the school buildings was closed for environmental concerns, the students were able to experience the epidemiological process in action. When an outbreak of shigella occurred in an elementary school, the students provided case follow-up in coordination with the local health department. When one of the teachers wanted to compare the use of traditional chairs versus ball chairs, nursing faculty provided consultation concerning the research process and students actively participated in that process.

EVALUATION

Limitations of the partnership include the time needed to establish relationships and develop trust within the district, numerous contacts and time necessary for coordination of activities, provision for support services, flexibility for working between the differing university and school district structure, management of time between university and school district responsibilities, and determination of how this position fits into the tenure/promotion process since it involves service learning.

This project has benefited both the University of Southern Colorado and Pueblo School District No. 60. It has emphasized the need for health care professional workers to guide district efforts to meet the students' health needs. It has developed a system of education and nursing delegation to support the efforts of nonhealth professionals in meeting schoolchildren's health needs. It has also expanded the community concept and practice arena in nursing education. Because of its success, neighboring school districts, which had previously rejected requests for provision of student experiences thinking them too time consuming, have now contacted the university to utilize nursing students in their school health programs.

This unique model is productive because of the collaboration between the school of nursing and the school district. Health needs of schoolchildren that were not being met are now being achieved. Nursing students experience firsthand community collaboration and practice. It indeed has met the mutual needs of the community and nursing education.

Index

Index